Question Bank
for
FINAL YEAR MBBS

Question Bank for FINAL YEAR MBBS (1990–2015)

Sanoob Sahabdeen MBBS
Sree Mookambika Institute of Medical Sciences
Kanyakumari, Tamil Nadu, India

Foreword
Singi Yatiraj

JAYPEE *The Health Sciences Publisher*
New Delhi | London | Philadelphia | Panama

JAYPEE **Jaypee Brothers Medical Publishers (P) Ltd**

Headquarters

Jaypee Brothers Medical Publishers (P) Ltd
4838/24, Ansari Road, Daryaganj
New Delhi 110 002, India
Phone: +91-11-43574357
Fax: +91-11-43574314
Email: jaypee@jaypeebrothers.com

Overseas Offices

J.P. Medical Ltd
83 Victoria Street, London
SW1H 0HW (UK)
Phone: +44 20 3170 8910
Fax: +44 (0)20 3008 6180
Email: info@jpmedpub.com

Jaypee-Highlights Medical Publishers Inc
City of Knowledge, Bld. 237, Clayton
Panama City, Panama
Phone: +1 507-301-0496
Fax: +1 507-301-0499
Email: cservice@jphmedical.com

Jaypee Medical Inc
325 Chestnut Street
Suite 412, Philadelphia, PA 19106, USA
Phone: +1 267-519-9789
Email: jpmed.us@gmail.com

Jaypee Brothers Medical Publishers (P) Ltd
17/1-B Babar Road, Block-B, Shaymali
Mohammadpur, Dhaka-1207
Bangladesh
Phone: +08801912003485
Email: jaypeedhaka@gmail.com

Jaypee Brothers Medical Publishers (P) Ltd
Bhotahity, Kathmandu, Nepal
Phone: +977-9741283608
Email: kathmandu@jaypeebrothers.com

Website: www.jaypeebrothers.com
Website: www.jaypeedigital.com

Inquiries for bulk sales may be solicited at: jaypee@jaypeebrothers.com

Question Bank for Final Year MBBS (1990–2015)

First Edition: **2016**

ISBN 978-93-5250-148-9

Printed at Rajkamal Electric Press, Plot No. 2, Phase-IV, Kundli, Haryana.

Dedicated to

My parents
My beloved sister & my family
My friends & my teachers
and
To the Almighty

FOREWORD

It is a matter of pride and honor to write the foreword for this book written by my student Dr Sanoob Sahabdeen in whom I am seeing a replica of me.

He has put in a great deal of effort and hard work in preparing this manuscript, that too, while he himself was in the final year. That speaks a lot about his character, self-determination and zeal to help others. He started out doing it free for his juniors in the college, but I personally felt such effort should help the masses and prompted him to release it as a book, which is in your hand, so it reaches and helps maximum number of students.

I am sure students will be benefited by this effort of Dr Sanoob. If you like this book and find it helpful, please do appreciate his hard work by mailing him. It keeps authors motivated.

I am sure he will soon come out with such books for other phases of MBBS.

Wishing him the best life and a grand success to this book and his future endeavors.

Singi Yatiraj
Associate Professor
Department of Forensic Medicine
Sree Mookambika Institute of Medical Sciences
Kanyakumari, Tamil Nadu, India

PREFACE

During my final year MBBS, I came to know that so far there were no question banks for final year MBBS, which covered The Tamil Nadu Dr MGR Medical University's previous year question papers. This made me to think of preparing a question bank, which covered the question papers of last 25 years (1990–2015) for all the subjects of final year MBBS. The Tamil Nadu Dr MGR Medical University question paper pattern has been changed from this academic year onwards, which has made it difficult for students to focus on important questions during their study leave. I hope this book will make things easier for them.

For this venture, I selected certain reputed textbooks, which are usually followed by students for examination preparations. From these books, I have selected one textbook for each subject and the questions have been arranged chapterwise with essay, short notes and short answers along with reference page numbers from the respective books. Page numbers from an additional textbook has also been given for all questions except for Medicine and Pediatrics. Questions that have appeared more recently and those repeated more than once have been marked along with the respective questions.

I have tried my level best in finding page numbers of answers from these textbooks. If any reader finds it to be incorrect or thinks it is better explained in other pages, please feel free to let me know through my email ID dr.sanoobsahabdeen@gmail.com and also do send your feedback.

Wishing you all the best for your upcoming examinations!

Good luck!!!

Sanoob Sahabdeen

ACKNOWLEDGMENTS

First of all I would like to thank Dr Singi Yatiraj, Associate Professor, Department of Forensic Medicine, Sree Mookambika Institute of Medical Sciences, Kanyakumari, Tamil Nadu, India, for giving me guidelines and helping me in publishing this book.

I would like to thank all my friends who gave me ideas and suggestions in making this book a reality and also to those who gave me their books for reference.

Expressions and emotions fail to find words to express thanks to my parents and family. I thank them for being a constant source of inspiration and motivation.

Also, I express my gratitude to Shri Jitendar P Vij (Group Chairman), Mr Ankit Vij (Group President), Mr Tarun Duneja (Director-Publishing) and Bengaluru Production Unit/Bengaluru Branch of M/s Jaypee Brothers Medical Publishers (P) Ltd, New Delhi, India, for publishing this book.

CONTENTS

Section 1

MEDICINE

Medicine

INSTRUCTIONS TO READERS

- Chapterwise based on Davidson's PRINCIPLES AND PRACTICE OF MEDICINE, 2nd edition (Code: DVDSN) with page numbers of answers
- The year in which questions have recently appeared (last nine question papers from Aug 2011 to Aug 2015) have been mentioned under the recent year's heading
- The number of times a question has been repeated, between 1990 and 2015, is mentioned within brackets along with the respective questions.

Chapters 1 to 12

1. Good Medical Practice
2. Therapeutics and Good Prescribing
3. Molecular and Genetic Factors in Disease
4. Immunological Factors in Disease
5. Environmental and Nutritional Factors in Disease
6. Principles of Infectious Disease
7. Ageing and Disease
8. Critical Illness
9. Poisoning
10. Medical Psychiatry
11. Oncology
12. Palliative Care and Pain

ESSAYS

	DVDSN	Recent Years
1. Write the causes, sequelae, investigations and management of obesity.	115	–
2. Discuss the causes of adult respiratory distress syndrome (ARDS), its pathophysiology and management.	192	–

3. Describe the approach to clinical recognition and initial therapy of psychiatric emergencies.	238	Feb 13
4. Discuss clinical features, diagnosis and management of mood disorders.	243	-
5. Define bipolar disorder. Discuss the etiology, clinical features and various mood disorders, and their management.	244, 243	Aug 15
6. Classify psychoses. Discuss clinical features, diagnosis and management of manic-depressive psychosis.	244	-
7. Define somatoform disorders. Discuss the etiology, clinical features of various somatoform disorders and their management.	245	Aug 14
8. Describe the clinical features, diagnosis and management of schizophrenia.	247	-
9. Clinical features, classification, diagnostic criteria and management of schizophrenia (2).	247	Feb 12, Aug 13
10. Discuss etiology, diagnosis and management of alcohol dependence. Add a note on delirium tremens.	252	-
11. Write in detail about the ill effects of chronic alcoholism, alcohol dependence and its management.	252	Feb 14
12. Define various personality disorders. Discuss the etiology, clinical features and management of personality disorders.	255	Feb 15

SHORT NOTES

1. Down syndrome.	56	Feb 12
2. Williams syndrome.	56	-
3. Regenerative medicine.	69	Feb 13
4. Immunoglobulin (Ig).	77	-
5. Cell-mediated immunity (CMI).	78	-
6. Steroid therapy.	90	-

7.	Anaphylaxis.	91	Aug 14
8.	Management of anaphylaxis.	92	Aug 13
9.	Smoking.	100	–
10.	Methods of smoking cessation.	101	Aug 13
11.	Thermoregulation.	103	–
12.	Heat stroke (2).	106	Feb 12, Aug 14
13.	Heat exhaustion.	106	–
14.	Polycythemia.	107, 271	–
15.	Drowning.	108	–
16.	Etiology of obesity and complications.	116	–
17.	Hypervitaminosis.	124	–
18.	Beriberi (2).	128	–
19.	Wernicke's encephalopathy (4).	128, 253	–
20.	Thiamine deficiency.	128	–
21.	Pellagra (6).	128	Aug 14
22.	Scurvy (2).	129	–
23.	Cretinism.	131, 755	–
24.	Rifampicin.	151	–
25.	Cephalosporins.	156	Aug 15
26.	Quinolones (2).	157	–
27.	Cause of falls in elderly.	172	–
28.	Delirium.	173	–
29.	Anaphylactic shock.	190	–
30.	ARDS (4).	192	–
31.	Management of septic shock.	201	–
32.	Gastric lavage (2).	210	–
33.	Acid poisoning.	210	Feb 15
34.	Paracetamol poisoning.	212	Aug 14
35.	Manifestations and management of digoxin toxicity.	215	Feb 14
36.	Drug abuse (2).	216	–
37.	Benzodiazepine poisoning.	217	Aug 13
38.	Management of carbon monoxide poisoning.	219	Feb 12

74.	Puerperal psychosis.	257	Aug 14
75.	Tumor marker.	270	–
76.	Oncological emergencies.	272	Feb 14
77.	Malignant pleural effusion.	275	Aug 14
78.	Hysteria.	–	–

SHORT ANSWERS

1.	Two side effects of calcium channel blockers.	26, 214	
2.	Four adverse effects of chloroquine.	26, 215	Feb 13
3.	List four drugs contraindicated in the first trimester of pregnancy.	37	–
4.	Cytokines.	74	–
5.	Name four cytokines.	74	Feb 12
6.	Acute phase reactants.	82	–
7.	Familial Mediterranean fever.	85	–
8.	Four immunosuppressive drugs.	96	Aug 13
9.	List four causes of hypothermia (2).	104	Feb 12, Aug 12
10.	Physiological effects of high altitude (acute motion sickness).	106	–
11.	Management of near-drowning patient.	108	–
12.	Name energy-yielding nutrients. Name the essential amino acids.	112, 114	–
13.	Mention four complications of obesity.	115	–
14.	Four causes of obesity.	116	Feb 12
15.	Name four endocrine causes of weight gain.	117	Feb 14
16.	List two important drugs used in the management of obesity.	119	Feb 15
17.	Four features of vitamin deficiencies.	124	Feb 13
18.	Pyridoxine.	129	–
19.	Mention three gram-negative bacilli.	136	–
20.	Risk factors for nosocomial infection.	146	–
21.	Name four groups of beta-lactam antibiotics.	154	Aug 14
22.	Third-generation cephalosporins.	156	–

23.	Name four macrolide antibiotics.	156	–
24.	Clinical uses of fluoroquinolones.	157	–
25.	List four adverse effects of dapsone.	158	Feb 12
26.	Four drugs used in fungal infection.	160	–
27.	Mention two changes in central nervous system (CNS) with aging and their corresponding consequences.	169	–
28.	Give two causes of delirium.	174	–
29.	List four causes for delirium in the elderly.	174	–
30.	Name four inotropic drugs.	191	Feb 13
31.	List four inotropic agents used for shock.	191	–
32.	Four causes of ARDS.	192	–
33.	List four complications of mechanical ventilation.	194	Feb 14
34.	Two indications for endotracheal intubation.	194	–
35.	List four causes of coma in a diabetic patient.	199	Aug 12
36.	List four dialyzable poisons.	211	Aug 13
37.	Management of barbiturate poisoning.	217	–
38.	List four causes of pinpoint pupils.	217, 221, 1172, 1177	Feb 12
39.	List four features of OPC poisoning.	220	Feb 13
40.	List two drugs in the management of OPC poisoning.	221	Aug 15
41.	Drugs used in organophosphate poisoning.	221	–
42.	Intermediate syndrome.	222	–
43.	Aluminum and zinc phosphide poisoning.	223	–
44.	Four clinical signs of snake bite.	226	Aug 12
45.	Enumerate four indications for antivenin administration.	227	–
46.	Name four complications of corrosive acid ingestion.	–	Feb 13
47.	Name four causes of acute confusional state.	238	Aug 12

48.	Obsessive-compulsive disorder.	243	–
49.	Psychosis.	248	–
50.	Any two phenothiazine group of drugs.	249	Feb 14
51.	Dementia.	250	–
52.	List four criteria for alcoholic dependence.	252	Aug 13
53.	List four features of neuropathic pain.	285	Aug 12
54.	Name four vaccines used in adults.	–	–
55.	List two vaccines for adult.	–	Feb 15
56.	Name four antitumor antibiotics.	–	Feb 12
57.	Ill effects of 'tobacco chewing'.	–	–
58.	Name four causes of metabolic encephalopathy.	–	Feb 14

Chapters 13 to 16

13. Infectious Disease
14. HIV* Infection and AIDS†
15. Sexually Transmitted Infections
16. Clinical Biochemistry and Metabolism

ESSAYS

	DVDSN	Recent Years
1. How will you record the normal body temperature at the bedside? What are the precautions to avoid mistakes? Discuss the differential diagnosis of fever with eruptions.	296	–
2. What are the causes of prolonged fever and its diagnostic approach in an adult.	–	–
3. Discuss the causes, clinical features, investigations and management of acute gastroenteritis.	306	–
4. Discuss the etiology, clinical features, laboratory diagnosis, management and complications of infectious mononucleosis.	320	Aug 14
5. What are the causes of thrombocytopenia? Discuss the clinical features and management of dengue fever.	1007, 322	–
6. Describe the etiology, clinical features and management of different types of dengue fever.	322	–
7. Describe clinical features, diagnosis and management of dengue fever. Write a note on complications and methods of prevention (3).	322	Aug 13
8. Elaborate on the etiopathogenesis, clinical features, laboratory diagnosis,		

*HIV, human immunodeficiency syndrome; †AIDS, acquired immunodeficiency syndrome.

	management and complications of dengue fever.	322	Aug 15
9.	Discuss the pathogenesis, clinical features, investigations, complications and management of leptospirosis (2).	336	–
10.	Etiology, clinical features, diagnosis, complications, investigations and management of enteric fever (4).	339	Aug 13
11.	Outline the life cycle of *Entamoeba histolytica*. Describe the etiopathogenesis, clinical features, management and prevention of amoebic dysentery. Add a note on its complications.	367	–
12.	Enumerate the causes, complication and management of HIV. Add a note on antiretroviral (ARV) drugs.	387	–
13.	Describe the clinical features, laboratory diagnosis, complications and management of HIV disease (2).	387	Feb 15
14.	Discuss the etiology, pathology, clinical features, opportunistic infections and treatment of AIDS.	387	–

SHORT NOTES

1.	Fever with rigor.	296	–
2.	Causes and management of hyperpyrexia.	296	–
3.	Oral rehydration therapy.	307	–
4.	Tropical eosinophilia (4).	311	–
5.	Subacute sclerosing panencephalitis.	314, 1207	Aug 13
6.	Congenital rubella syndrome (CRS).	315	–
7.	Shingles.	318	–
8.	Herpes zoster (2).	318	–
9.	Complications of mumps.	319	–
10.	Swine flu (2).	320	–
11.	Infectious mononucleosis.	320	–
12.	Dengue fever.	322	–
13.	Dengue shock syndrome.	322	Feb 12

14.	Herpes simplex (2).	325	–
15.	Chikungunya fever.	329	Aug 14
16.	Brucellosis.	333	–
17.	Leptospirosis (2).	336	Aug 12
18.	Weil's disease (3).	337	–
19.	Weil's syndrome.	337	Feb 14
20.	Clinical features of plague.	338	–
21.	Enteric fever (4).	339	Feb 13, Feb 15
22.	Food poisoning.	341	–
23.	Cholera.	344	Aug 14
24.	Treatment of lepromatous leprosy.	348	–
25.	Polyneuritic leprosy.	349	–
26.	Erythema nodosum leprosum (ENL).	349	–
27.	Lepra reaction (6).	349	–
28.	Chemotherapy of leprosy.	349	–
29.	Tropical splenomegaly.	355	–
30.	Cerebral malaria (4).	355	–
31.	Treatment of cerebral malaria (2).	357	–
32.	Chemoprophylaxis of malaria.	357	Aug 15
33.	Extraintestinal amebiasis.	367	–
34.	Amebic dysentery.	367	–
35.	Hookworm disease.	369	–
36.	Casoni test.	–	–
37.	Bancroftian filariasis.	372	–
38.	Liver flukes.	378, 312, 266	Aug 15
39.	Hydatid disease.	380	–
40.	Mucormycosis.	384	–
41.	CD4 count.	393	–
42.	AIDS.	395	–
43.	Opportunistic HIV infection.	395	–
44.	Pulmonary complications of HIV infection.	400	–
45.	Treatment of AIDS.	407	–
46.	Zidovudine.	407	–

47.	Highly active antiretroviral therapy (HAART) principles (2).	407	–
48.	Postexposure prophylaxis of HIV.	410	Aug 14
49.	Lymphogranuloma venereum (LGV).	424	–
50.	Potassium-sparing diuretics.	435	–
51.	Hyponatremia.	437	–
52.	Syndrome of inappropriate antidiuretic hormone secretion (SIADH).	438	–
53.	Hyperkalemia (4).	442	–
54.	Treatment of hyperkalemia.	442	Aug 13
55.	Metabolic acidosis.	445	–
56.	Tumor lysis syndrome.	449	Feb 14
57.	HMG-CoA reductase inhibitors.	456	Aug 13

SHORT ANSWERS

1.	List four causes of fever and rash.	295	Feb 12
2.	Enumerate four causes for infective diarrhea.	306	–
3.	Oral rehydration therapy.	307	–
4.	Name the ingredients in the oral rehydration salts (ORS).	307	Feb 12
5.	Four complications of measles.	314	Feb 14
6.	Four complications of chickenpox.	317	–
7.	Herpes zoster (2).	318	–
8.	List four antiherpes virus agents.	318	Aug 13
9.	Four features of swine flu.	320	Feb 13
10.	List two ways of transmission of ebola virus diseases.	325	Feb 15
11.	List two major clinical features of ebola virus disease.	325	Aug 15
12.	Prion diseases.	329	–
13.	Four causes of fever with jaundice (3).	337, 355, 948	Aug 12, Feb 12, Aug 13
14.	Name any four antibiotics used in the treatment of enteric fever.	340	Aug 12

15.	*Clostridium difficile.*	343	–
16.	Lepra reaction.	349	Feb 14
17.	Name four clinical conditions for use of rifampicin.	350, 352, 694	Feb 12
18.	Four common features of falciparum malaria.	355	–
19.	Enumerate four manifestations/ complications of severe falciparum malaria.	357	–
20.	Name four complications of falciparum malaria.	357	Aug 12
21.	Drugs for amebiasis.	368	Aug 13
22.	Mention four AIDS-defining diseases.	395	–
23.	List four common opportunistic infections seen in HIV-infected patients.	395	–
24.	Name four opportunistic infections in AIDS, if CD4 count < 50.	395	Aug 13
25.	List four cutaneous manifestations of HIV/AIDS.	397	Aug 13
26.	Four causes of oral ulcerations.	398, 1111, 1119	–
27.	Neuropsychiatric manifestations of AIDS.	402	Aug 12
28.	Name four antiretroviral drugs.	407	–
29.	List the five categories of drugs used in HIV treatment.	407	Aug 14
30.	Postexposure prophylaxis in HIV infection.	410	–
31.	Name four sexually transmitted infections presenting as genital ulcers.	415	–
32.	Name four sexually transmitted diseases (STDs).	419	Feb 13
33.	Name the TORCH organisms.	–	–

Chapter 17

17. Kidney and Urinary Tract Disease

ESSAYS

	DVDSN	Recent Years
1. Describe the clinical features, complications and management of nephritic syndrome (2).	475, 497	–
2. Describe the etiology, clinical features, differential diagnosis, diagnosis and management of nephrotic syndrome (2).	476	–
3. Mention etiology, clinical features, investigations and management of acute renal failure (ARF).	478	–
4. List five causes of ARF. Discuss the pathophysiology and management of acute tubular necrosis.	479	–
5. What are the causes of ARF? Discuss the etiopathogenesis, clinical features and management of acute glomerulonephritis (3).	479, 498	Aug 12
6. Describe the clinical features of chronic renal failure. Outline the pathogenesis of renal osteodystrophy. Mention the reversible factors in chronic renal failure (CRF).	484	–
7. Describe the etiopathogenesis, clinical features, complications, investigations and management of CRF (2).	484	–
8. Discuss etiology, clinical evaluation and management of urinary tract infection (UTI). Add a note on recurrent UTI.	511	–

SHORT NOTES

1.	Endocrine function of kidney.	464	–
2.	Microscopic urinary sediments.	468	–
3.	Urine examination.	468	–
4.	Polyuria.	472	–
5.	Erectile impotence.	474	–
6.	Sexual dysfunction.	474	–
7.	Hematuria.	474	–
8.	How to evaluate a case of hematuria?	474	Aug 13
9.	Proteinuria.	476	–
10.	Nephrotic syndrome (5).	476	Aug 12
11.	Acute renal failure.	478	Feb 15
12.	ARF and CRF.	478, 483	–
13.	Etiology and treatment of ARF.	478	–
14.	Renal osteodystrophy.	486	–
15.	Renal replacement therapy.	488	–
16.	Hemodialysis.	489, 490	–
17.	Lupus nephritis.	500	Aug 15
18.	Poststreptococcal glomerulonephritis (PSGN).	501	–
19.	Alport's syndrome (3).	502	Aug 14
20.	Polycystic kidney disease.	505	Aug 14
21.	Urinary tract infection.	511	Feb 14
22.	Classification and treatment of pyelonephritis.	513	–

SHORT ANSWERS

1.	Causes of hematuria (2).	475	–
2.	Microalbuminuria.	476	–
3.	List four causes of microalbuminuria.	476	Feb 12
4.	Four features of nephrotic syndrome (2).	477	–
5.	List two causes of unilateral limb edema.	478	Aug 15
6.	Two causes of acute kidney injury.	479	–
7.	Four cardinal features of renal failure.	479	Feb 12

8.	List four important causes of end-stage renal failure.	484	Aug 14
9.	Four indications for dialysis (renal).	491, 211	–
10.	Four clinical features of glomerular disease.	498	–
11.	Four cardinal features of glomerulonephritis.	498	Feb 13
12.	List two important causes of nephrolithiasis.	507	Feb 15
13.	List two causes of ureteric stones.	507	Aug 15
14.	Four predisposing factors for renal stones.	507	–
15.	Four organisms causing UTI.	512	–
16.	Investigation of patient with UTI.	512	–
17.	Four complications of urinary catheterization.	513	Feb 13
18.	Triad of renal cell carcinoma.	516	Aug 13

Chapter 18

18. Cardiovascular Disease

ESSAYS

	DVDSN	Recent Years
1. A 40-year-old obese male, a chronic smoker and an alcoholic, reports to you with retrosternal discomfort. Discuss your approach towards diagnosis and management.	539	–
2. What are the causes of acute chest pain in a 40-year-old man? Describe the clinical features, electrocardiogram (ECG) changes, biochemical markers and management of acute myocardial infarction.	541, 589	Aug 12
3. Describe the types, clinical features, complications and management of heart failure.	546	–
4. Define and classify heart failure. Discuss the clinical assessment of heart failure with investigations and management of congestive cardiac failure.	546	–
5. Define heart failure. Discuss pathophysiology and classification of heart failure. Outline the management of chronic heart failure.	546	–
6. What are the precipitating factors for heart failure? What are the investigations available to assess coronary artery disease?	548, 583	–
7. Discuss the etiology, clinical features, complications and management of atrial fibrillation.	564	–
8. Mention the causes, signs and symptoms, diagnosis and treatment of complete heart block.	572	–

9.	Discuss pathophysiology, clinical features and complications of acute myocardial infarction. Add a note on thrombolytic therapy.	589	–
10.	Discuss the risk factors, clinical features, complications, investigations and management of acute myocardial infarction (3).	589	–
11.	Explain in detail about the clinical features, investigations and management of acute coronary syndrome with particular reference to myocardial infarction.	589	Feb 14
12.	What are the complications of acute myocardial infarction? Define cardiogenic shock and outline its management.	596, 544	–
13.	Discuss the etiology, clinical features, investigations and management of essential hypertension.	607	–
14.	Discuss the etiology, complication and management of systemic hypertension.	607	–
15.	Define, classify and discuss in detail about management of hypertension.	607	–
16.	Discuss the pathogenesis, clinical features and treatment of acute rheumatic fever.	614	–
17.	Mention clinical features of rheumatic carditis. Discuss investigations, management and prophylaxis of rheumatic heart disease.	614	–
18.	Mention clinical features of infective endocarditis. Discuss investigations, management and prophylaxis of infective endocarditis.	625	–
19.	Discuss etiology, clinical features, investigations and management of infective endocarditis.	625	Aug 12
20.	Describe the etiology, clinical features, diagnosis and management of subacute bacterial endocarditis.	625	–
21.	Outline the general clinical features of cyanotic congenital heart disease.		

	Question	Page	Exam
	What are the clinical features and management of patent ductus arteriosus? Write a note on Eisenmenger's syndrome.	629	–
22.	Discuss the etiology, clinical features, diagnosis and management of pericardial effusion.	640	–
23.	Discuss the etiology, clinical features, diagnosis, investigations and management of pericardial effusion. Add a note on cardiac tamponade (2).	640	Feb 12

SHORT NOTES

	Question	Page	Exam
1.	Normal and abnormal jugular venous pulsations.	527, 624, 724	–
2.	Cardiac enzymes.	535, 593	Aug 13
3.	Chest pain.	539	–
4.	Pulsus alternans.	545	–
5.	Third heart sound (S3) gallop.	548	–
6.	Acute cor pulmonale.	548	–
7.	Afterload reduction in chronic cardiac failure.	550	–
8.	Cardiopulmonary resuscitation.	558	Aug 12, Feb 13
9.	Advanced life support.	558	Aug 14
10.	Cardiac arrest management.	558	–
11.	Atrial fibrillation (3).	564	Feb 13
12.	Clinical signs and treatment of atrial fibrillation.	564	Aug 12
13.	Supraventricular tachycardia (SVT).	567	–
14.	Torsades de pointes.	570	–
15.	Antiarrhythmic drugs and doses.	575	–
16.	Unstable angina (2).	589	–
17.	Management of acute myocardial infarction (MI).	593	–
18.	Thrombolytic agents used in MI.	594	Aug 15
19.	Thrombolytic treatment in acute MI.	594	–

20.	Mechanical complications of MI.	597	Feb 15
21.	Dressler's syndrome.	597	Aug 14
22.	Left ventricle (LV) systolic function.	598	–
23.	Methods and mistakes of recording blood pressure.	608	–
24.	Outline pharmacotherapy of hypertension.	611	–
25.	Hypertensive emergencies.	612	Feb 12
26.	Acute rheumatic fever.	614	–
27.	Rheumatic fever prophylaxis.	615	Feb 13
28.	X-ray and ECG findings in mitral stenosis (MS).	617	–
29.	Water hammer pulse.	623	–
30.	Tricuspid regurgitation.	624	–
31.	Infective endocarditis (3).	625	Feb 14
32.	Modified Duke criteria.	627	–
33.	Eisenmenger's syndrome.	631	Feb 14
34.	Central cyanosis.	631	–
35.	Cyanosis.	631	Aug 12
36.	Patent ductus arteriosus (PDA).	631	–
37.	Atrial septal defect.	632	Aug 14
38.	Coarctation of aorta.	632	Aug 12, Feb 14
39.	Ventricular septal defect (VSD).	633	–
40.	Tetralogy of Fallot (2).	634	–
41.	Cardiomyopathy.	636	Feb 15
42.	Paradoxical pulse.	640	–
43.	Pericardial effusion.	640	–
44.	Cardiac tamponade.	640	Aug 14
45.	Angiotensin-converting enzyme (ACE) inhibitors (3).	26, 176, 522, 551, 599, 611	–
46.	Calcium channel blockers.	26, 214, 586, 612, 618, 638	–
47.	Beta blockers.	26, 176, 552, 574, 586, 599 604, 667, 946	–

48. Indications and contraindications of beta blockers.	552, 574, 586, 599, 604, 667, 946	Aug 12

SHORT ANSWERS

1. Four causes of acute pulmonary edema.	482, 494, 597, 714	Feb 12
2. List four causes of high volume collapsing pulse.	527	Aug 12
3. Name four cardiac enzymes.	535, 593	Feb 13
4. List four important signs of cardiac failure.	549	Aug 14
5. Four drugs used in heart failure.	550	Feb 12
6. Mention drugs used in acute pulmonary edema.	550	-
7. Four causes of syncope.	554	Feb 13
8. Causes of bradycardia.	563	-
9. Name four beta blockers.	574	Aug 14
10. List four drugs used for treatment of chronic stable angina.	585	-
11. List four major contraindications of thrombolytic therapy.	596	Feb 14
12. Four causes of secondary hypertension (2).	607	-
13. Name the four target organs of hypertension.	608	Aug 12
14. Features of hypertensive encephalopathy.	609	Feb 12
15. List four antihypertensive drugs.	611	-
16. Name two parenteral antihypertensive drug.	612	Feb 15
17. List four contraindications for ACE inhibitors.	613, 971	Feb 12
18. Two contraindications to beta blockers.	613	-
19. Angiotensin receptor blockers indications.	613	-
20. Enumerate the major criteria of rheumatic fever.	614	Feb 14

21.	Four features of Jones criteria.	614	–
22.	List four major Jones criteria for rheumatic fever.	614	Aug 13
23.	List two causes of elevated antistreptolysin O (ASO) titer.	615	Aug 15
24.	Auscultatory signs of MS.	616	–
25.	List two important signs of infective endocarditis.	626	Aug 15
26.	List four causes of central cyanosis.	631	Feb 14
27.	Four causes of dilated cardiomyopathy.	636	Aug 13

Chapter 19

19. Respiratory Disease

ESSAYS

	DVDSN	Recent Years
1. Compare the clinical features of pleural effusion, hydropneumothorax, consolidation and cavity.	645	–
2. Discuss the etiology, clinical features and differential diagnosis of pulmonary fibrosis.	645, 707, 712	–
3. Mention the causes of hemoptysis. Describe in detail the current trends in management of pulmonary tuberculosis (TB).	659, 693	–
4. How will you diagnose pleural effusion? What are the causes? Discuss briefly the management of one of them.	661	–
5. What are the common causes of pleural effusion? Describe the clinical features, diagnosis and management of tubercular pleural effusion.	661, 688	–
6. Discuss the signs, symptoms and management of right-sided tuberculous pleural effusion.	661, 688	–
7. Write in detail about the underlying causes, blood gas abnormalities in type I and type II respiratory failure, and management of both conditions.	663	–
8. Describe the pathophysiology, clinical features, investigations, complications and management of acute severe asthma.	666	–
9. Define bronchial asthma. Write in detail the etiopathogenesis, clinical features and management of bronchial asthma (2).	666	–

10. Mention the conditions producing wheeze in the lungs. How do you clinically identify them? Detail the treatment of status asthmaticus (3).	666	-
11. Discuss etiology, pathophysiology, clinical features and management of chronic obstructive pulmonary disease (COPD) (2).	673	-
12. Discuss the etiology, pathology, clinical features, investigations and management of chronic bronchitis.	673	Feb 14
13. Discuss the etiopathogenesis, clinical features, diagnosis, complications and treatment of bronchiectasis.	678	-
14. Discuss the etiology, clinical features, complications and management of cystic fibrosis of lung.	680	-
15. Discuss the etiology, clinical features, diagnosis, complications and management of lobar pneumonia.	682	-
16. Define pneumonia. Discuss the clinical features, investigations, differential diagnosis and management of community-acquired pneumonia (2).	682	-
17. Discuss the pathology, clinical features, investigations, complications and management of pneumococcal pneumonia.	682	-
18. Classify pneumonias. Describe the clinical features. Mention the role of bronchoscopy in the diagnosis and treatment of respiratory disorders.	682, 651	-
19. Describe in detail the causes, clinical features and management of pneumonia.	682	Feb 13
20. Discuss pathology, clinical evaluation and management of pulmonary tuberculosis. Add a note on TB in patients with HIV infection.	688, 400	-
21. Discuss the etiology, clinical features, investigations and treatment of tropical pulmonary eosinophilia.	713	-

22.	Discuss the etiology, pathophysiology, clinical features, prevention, investigations and management of acute pulmonary embolism (3).	721	-
23.	Describe the etiology, types, clinical features, investigations and management of pneumothorax (2).	728	-

SHORT NOTES

1.	Pulmonary function test (PFT).	652	-
2.	Spirometry.	652, 668, 675	Feb 13
3.	Sputum examination.	652	-
4.	Arterial blood gases.	653	-
5.	Acute pulmonary edema.	658	Aug 15
6.	Hemoptysis with scanty clinicoradiological findings.	658	-
7.	Hemoptysis—management.	659	-
8.	Pleural effusion.	661	-
9.	Chylothorax.	661	-
10.	Diagnostic pleural aspiration and biopsy.	661	-
11.	Acute severe asthma.	666	Feb 12
12.	Bronchial asthma—step wise management.	669	Aug 15
13.	Management of acute severe bronchial asthma (3).	671	Aug 12
14.	Status asthmaticus.	671	-
15.	Emphysema.	673	-
16.	Management of COPD.	675	Feb 12
17.	Dry bronchiectasis.	678	-
18.	Community-acquired pneumonia.	682	Feb 14
19.	Hospital-acquired pneumonia.	685	-
20.	Lung abscess.	687	Aug 12, Feb 13
21.	*Pneumocystis jiroveci* pneumonia.	688	-
22.	Interpretation of Mantoux test.	695	-

23.	Directly observed treatment, short-course (DOTS).	695	–
24.	Drug-resistant tuberculosis.	696	Feb 12
25.	Multidrug-resistant tuberculosis (MDR-TB) (2).	696	Aug 13
26.	Atypical mycobacteria.	696	Feb 13
27.	Aspergillosis.	697	–
28.	Non-metastatic extrapulmonary manifestations of bronchogenic carcinoma.	702	–
29.	Pulmonary eosinophilia (2).	713	–
30.	Tropical pulmonary eosinophilia.	713	–
31.	Coal worker's pneumoconiosis.	716	–
32.	Asbestosis.	718	Aug 13
33.	D-dimer.	722	–
34.	Pneumothorax.	728	Feb 15

SHORT ANSWERS

1.	Mention four types of breathing patterns.	–	Aug 13
2.	Four pulmonary function tests.	652	–
3.	Four causes of hemoptysis (2).	659	–
4.	Two causes of milky pleural fluid.	662	–
5.	Name four precipitating factors for asthma.	666	Feb 13
6.	List two systemic manifestations of COPD.	673	Feb 15
7.	List four causes of bronchiectasis.	678	Aug 12
8.	Two causes of cavities in lung.	678	–
9.	List four external markers of TB.	690	Aug 14
10.	Non-pulmonary complications of pulmonary TB.	690	–
11.	Four drugs used in chemotherapy of TB.	694	–
12.	DOTS therapy (2).	695	–
13.	Four drugs used in MDR-TB (2).	696	–
14.	Any two second-line antitubercular (ATT) drugs.	–	Feb 14
15.	Four second-line ATT drugs.	–	–
16.	Anticyclic citrullinated peptides (CCP) antibody.	708	–

17.	List two causes of pulmonary embolism.	721	Feb 15
18.	List four important risk factors of venous thromboembolism.	721	Aug 14
19.	List two important signs of pulmonary hypertension.	724	Feb 15
20.	List four causes of pneumothorax.	728	Feb 14
21.	Mention types of bronchial breath sounds.	–	–

Chapters 20 and 21

20. Endocrine Disease 21. Diabetes Mellitus

ESSAYS

	DVDSN	Recent Years
1. Discuss the etiology, clinical features, investigations and management of hyperthyroidism.	740	-
2. Discuss etiology, clinical assessment and management of hypothyroidism. Add a note on myxedema coma.	743	-
3. Mention the etiology, diagnosis, complications and treatment of hypothyroidism.	743	-
4. Discuss etiology, clinical features, investigations and management of adrenal insufficiency.	777	-
5. Discuss the etiopathogenesis of insulin-dependent diabetes mellitus (IDDM) and non-insulin-dependent diabetes mellitus (NIDDM). Briefly discuss etiopathogenesis of diabetic ketoacidosis (DKA) and its management.	802, 811	-
6. Describe the etiopathogenesis, clinical features and management of diabetes mellitus (DM) (2).	802	-
7. Classify DM. Enumerate the chronic complications of DM. How would you treat and monitor the control in uncomplicated type II diabetes?	807, 826, 820	-
8. Classify DM. Enumerate the acute complications of DM. Define about Dawn and Somogyi phenomenon.	807, 826	Aug 13

9.	Diagnostic criteria of DM. Elaborate on the clinical features and management of DKA.	809, 811	Aug15
10.	Describe the clinical features, investigations, complications and management of DKA (2).	811	–

SHORT NOTES

1.	Thyroid function tests.	739	Feb 14
2.	Thyroid profile.	739	–
3.	Diagnosis and complications of thyrotoxicosis.	740	–
4.	Thyroid storm.	742	Feb 12
5.	Myxedema madness.	745	–
6.	Myxedema coma.	745	–
7.	Graves' disease.	747	Feb 14
8.	Agranulocytosis (3).	749, 694	–
9.	Hirsutism.	763	–
10.	Klinefelter's syndrome.	766	–
11.	Tetany (3).	768	–
12.	Pseudohypoparathyroidism.	770	–
13.	Cushing syndrome.	773	Aug 12, Feb 13
14.	Addison's disease (4).	777	–
15.	Classification of adrenal insufficiency.	777	–
16.	Addison's crisis.	779	Feb 12
17.	Adrenal crisis.	779	–
18.	Insulinoma.	785	–
19.	Sheehan's syndrome.	787, 789	–
20.	Acromegaly (2).	792	Aug 12
21.	Diabetes insipidus.	794	–
22.	Metabolic syndrome.	805	Aug 13
23.	Classification of DM.	807	Feb 14
24.	Glycosylated hemoglobin.	808	–
25.	Oral glucose tolerance test.	809	–
26.	Diabetic ketoacidosis (4).	811	–

27.	Management of DKA.	813	–
28.	Hypoglycemia (2).	814	–
29.	Non-ketotic hyperosmolar diabetic coma.	814	–
30.	Hyperosmolar non-ketotic state.	814	Feb 13
31.	Drug-induced hypoglycemia.	814	–
32.	Oral hypoglycemic drugs (2).	821	–
33.	Alpha-glucosidase inhibitors.	823	Feb 12, Aug 14
34.	Sitagliptin.	824	Feb 15
35.	Insulin therapy.	824	–
36.	Insulin glargine.	824	Aug 15
37.	Insulin analogues.	824	–
38.	Newer insulin.	825	–
39.	Diabetic retinopathy.	828	Feb 14
40.	Diabetic nephropathy.	830	Feb 15
41.	Diabetes herpetiformis.	–	–
42.	Causes of secondary diabetes.	–	–
43.	Brittle diabetes.	–	–

SHORT ANSWERS

1.	Name four counterregulatory hormones.	736	Feb 12
2.	Four symptoms of thyrotoxicosis.	741	Feb 13
3.	Drugs used in hyperthyroidism.	741	–
4.	Four symptoms of myxedema.	745	Feb 12
5.	List two important causes of thyroid swelling.	746	Feb 15
6.	List four important signs of Grave's ophthalmopathy.	750	Aug 14
7.	Two causes of non-pitting pedal edema (2).	751	–
8.	Four drugs causing gynecomastia (2).	762	Aug 13
9.	Name four causes of gynecomastia.	762	Aug 12
10.	Polycystic ovarian syndrome.	764	–
11.	Name four signs of hypocalcemia.	768	Aug 12
12.	Mention four causes of adrenocortical insufficiency.	777	–

13.	Whipple's triad in hypoglycemia.	783	Aug 13
14.	Four clinical features of carcinoid tumors.	784	–
15.	Four clinical features of gigantism.	792	Feb 12
16.	Four clinical features of acromegaly.	792	Feb 13
17.	World Health Organization (WHO) criteria for diagnosis of DM.	809	–
18.	List four metabolic/biochemical features of DKA.	812	–
19.	Four signs of DKA.	812	–
20.	List four causes for hypoglycemia.	815	–
21.	Four neuroglycopenic symptoms of hypoglycemia.	815	–
22.	List four features of hypoglycemia.	815	Aug 14
23.	Four risk factors of gestational DM.	817	–
24.	Mention oral hypoglycemic agents.	821	–
25.	List four newer drugs in the management of type 2 DM.	821	Aug 14
26.	Incretin mimetics.	823	Aug 12
27.	Mention four complications of DM.	826	–
28.	List four important features of diabetic retinopathy.	828	Aug 14

Chapters 22 and 23

22. Alimentary Disease and Pancreatic Disease
23. Liver and Biliary Tract Disease

ESSAYS

	DVDSN	Recent Years
1. Discuss the etiology, clinical features, diagnosis, complications and management of chronic peptic ulcer.	872	-
2. Discuss the etiology, clinical features, diagnosis and management of acute pancreátitis (2).	889	-
3. Discuss the etiopathogenesis, clinical features, diagnosis and management of inflammatory bowel disease.	897	-
4. Discuss the pathogenesis, clinical features, investigations and management of ulcerative colitis.	897	-
5. Discuss the causes, clinical features, investigations and management of ascites.	938	-
6. Describe etiopathogenesis, clinical features, complications, investigations and management of hepatic encephalopathy (2).	941	Aug 12
7. Enumerate the causes of cirrhosis of liver. Discuss the clinical features, investigations and complications of alcoholic cirrhosis of liver. Write briefly the management strategy of hepatic encephalopathy.	942, 957, 941	-
8. Discuss the etiology, pathology, clinical features, complications and management of postnecrotic cirrhosis of liver.	-	-
9. Discuss the etiology, clinical features and management of portal hypertension.	945	-
10. Classify viral hepatitis. Describe the clinical features, natural history, management and prophylaxis of hepatitis.	948	-

11.	Describe the etiopathogenesis, clinical features, investigations and treatment of viral hepatitis. Add a note on prevention (2).	948	Feb 12

SHORT NOTES

1.	Upper gastrointestinal (UGI) endoscopy.	846	Feb 13
2.	Lower gastrointestinal (LGI) bleed.	856	–
3.	Marked loss of weight.	859	–
4.	Gastroesophageal reflux disease (GERD).	865	–
5.	Proton pump inhibitor (PPI) (2).	867	–
6.	Omeprazole.	867	–
7.	*Helicobacter pylori (H. pylori).*	872	–
8.	Peptic ulcer disease complications.	875	–
9.	Zollinger-Ellison syndrome (2).	876	Feb 14
10.	Celiac disease.	880	–
11.	Malabsorption syndrome (3).	880	Feb 13
12.	Tropical sprue.	882	–
13.	Treatment of acute pancreatitis.	892	Feb 14
14.	Ulcerative colitis.	897	Feb 13
15.	Irritable bowel syndrome (4).	907	Feb 14
16.	Liver function tests (LFTs).	928	–
17.	Techniques of liver biopsy (2).	931	–
18.	Fulminant hepatic failure.	932	–
19.	Hemolytic jaundice.	936	–
20.	Refractory ascites.	940	–
21.	Hepatorenal syndrome.	940	Aug 13
22.	Management of ascites.	940	–
23.	Spontaneous bacterial peritonitis (2).	941	–
24.	Management of hepatic encephalopathy (3).	942	–
25.	Portal hypertension.	945	–
26.	Management of acute bleeding from esophageal varices.	946	–
27.	Hepatitis B management.	952	–
28.	Hepatitis C virus.	954	–
29.	Hepatitis C.	954	Feb 15

30.	Hydatid cyst.	956	Feb 15
31.	Amebic liver abscess.	957	Aug 14
32.	Alcoholic liver disease.	957	–
33.	Hepatoma.	967	–
34.	Wilson's disease.	973	Aug 13

SHORT ANSWERS

1.	Mention two indications and two contraindications for UGI endoscopy.	848	–
2.	Four complications of UGI endoscopy.	848	–
3.	List four causes of UGI bleed.	853	Aug 13
4.	List four causes of parotid gland swelling.	864	Aug 14
5.	List any four methods for the diagnosis of *H. pylori* infection.	873	Aug 12, Aug 13
6.	Eradication of *H. pylori.*	874	–
7.	Drugs in *H. pylori.*	874	–
8.	List four important risk factors for gastric cancer.	878	Aug 14
9.	Four drugs used in ulcerative colitis.	903	–
10.	Mention four LFTs used to assess liver disease.	928	–
11.	List four congenital hyperbilirubinemia disorders.	937	Feb 12
12.	Four causes of obstructive jaundice.	937	Feb 13
13.	Charcot's triad.	938	–
14.	Hemorrhagic ascites.	939	–
15.	Name four precipitating factors for hepatic encephalopathy.	941	Feb 12
16.	List four non-respiratory causes of clubbing.	943	Aug 14
17.	Two complications of portal hypertension.	945	–
18.	Acute viral hepatitis.	948	–
19.	List four drugs used in chronic hepatitis B.	953	Aug 14
20.	List the schedule of hepatitis B vaccination.	–	Aug 15
21.	Two causes of liver abscess.	956	–

22.	Four poor prognostic factors in alcoholic liver disease.	959	–
23.	Four causes of pruritus without skin disease.	963, 966, 272	–
24.	Name four hepatotoxic drugs.	971	Feb 12
25.	Name four PPIs (2).	–	Feb 12

Chapter 24

24. Blood Disease

ESSAYS

	DVDSN	Recent Years
1. Describe the different blood groups, techniques and implications of blood transfusion. Mention the diseases transmitted through blood transfusion.	1011	–
2. Mention the medical indications of blood transfusion. What are the contraindications? Discuss briefly the measures you would take to avoid hazards of blood transfusion.	1011	–
3. Describe the etiology, pathophysiology, blood picture, clinical features, investigations and principles of management of iron-deficiency anemia (2).	1021	–
4. Discuss the prevalence, complications and management of iron-deficiency anemia (4).	1021	Feb 12
5. Mention the role of erythropoietic substances. Describe the clinical manifestations, diagnosis and treatment of megaloblastic anemia.	992, 1024	–
6. Describe the pathology, clinical features, investigations and management of sickle cell anemia.	1032	–
7. Classify acute myeloid leukemia (AML). Describe the etiopathogenesis, diagnosis and management of acute myeloid leukemia.	1036	–
8. Discuss the etiology, natural history, clinical features, investigation and management of chronic myeloid leukemia (CML).	1039	–
9. Discuss etiopathogenesis, clinical features, investigations and management of non-Hodgkin's lymphoma.	1043	–

10.	Define aplastic anemia. Discuss the etiology, clinical features, investigations and treatment of aplastic anemia.	1048	Feb 14
11.	Mention the common bleeding disorders. Discuss in detail any one of them.	1049	Feb 13

SHORT NOTES

1.	Splenomegaly (2).	1006	–
2.	Blood component therapy.	1011	Feb 12
3.	Hazards of blood transfusion.	1012	Feb 12
4.	Bone marrow transplantation.	1017	–
5.	Allogeneic bone marrow transplant.	1017	–
6.	Low-molecular-weight (LMW) heparin.	1018	–
7.	Iron-deficiency anemia.	1021	Feb 13, Feb 14, Aug 12
8.	Parenteral iron therapy.	1023	–
9.	Megaloblastic anemia (2).	1024	–
10.	Pernicious anemia (2).	1025	–
11.	Schilling test.	1025	–
12.	Laboratory evaluation of hemolysis.	1026	–
13.	Laboratory diagnosis of hemolytic anemia.	1026	–
14.	Sideroblastic anemia (3).	–	–
15.	Sickle cell disease.	1032	–
16.	Clinical features of sickle cell anemia.	1032	–
17.	Management of thalassemias.	1034	Feb 12
18.	AML.	1036	–
19.	Management of acute leukemia.	1036	Aug 12
20.	CML.	1039	–
21.	CML—investigations and complications (2).	1039	–
22.	Lymphoma.	1041	–
23.	Hodgkin's lymphoma.	1042	Aug 15
24.	Staging and management of Hodgkin's lymphoma.	1042	–

25.	Multiple myeloma.	1046	–
26.	Thalidomide.	1047, 1119, 349, 1223	–
27.	Aplastic anemia.	1048	–
28.	Laboratory diagnosis of aplastic anemia.	1048	–
29.	Polycythemia rubra vera (3).	1049	Feb 14
30.	Primary proliferative polycythemia.	1003, 1049	–
31.	Bleeding disorders.	1049	–
32.	Idiopathic thrombocytopenic purpura (ITP) (4).	1050	Aug 14
33.	Clinical and laboratory features of hemophilia.	1051	–
34.	Hemophilia (5).	1051	–
35.	von Willebrand's disease.	1053	–
36.	Disseminated intravascular coagulation (DIC) (2).	1055	–

SHORT ANSWERS

1.	List four important causes of eosinophilia (2).	1004	Aug 14
2.	Mention four causes for neutropenia.	1004	–
3.	Name four drugs causing neutropenia.	1005	–
4.	Four causes of generalized lymphadenopathy.	1005	–
5.	Four causes of massive splenomegaly (2).	1006	–
6.	Name four complications of blood transfusion.	1012	Aug 13
7.	Stem cell transplant.	1017	–
8.	Two indications for bone marrow transplantation.	1017	–
9.	List four indications for anticoagulation therapy.	1018	Aug 12
10.	Name two glycoprotein (GP) IIb/IIIa antagonists.	1019	–
11.	List four causes of megaloblastic anemia.	1024	–
12.	Blood picture of dimorphic anemia.	–	–

13. Mention four neurological features of B_{12} deficiency.	1024	–
14. List four features of vitamin B_{12} deficiency.	1024	Aug 12
15. Plasmapheresis.	–	–
16. Name four hemoglobinopathy.	1031	–
17. What is sickle cell crisis?	1032	–
18. List four diagnostic features of beta thalassemia.	1034	Aug 14
19. Importance of Philadelphia chromosome.	1039	–
20. Stages of Hodgkin's lymphoma.	1042	–
21. List four myeloproliferative diseases.	1048	Feb 12
22. List four causes for purpura.	1050, 1056, 1119, 1304	Aug 12

Chapters 25 to 27

ESSAYS

	DVDSN	Recent Years
1. Discuss the etiology, pathogenesis, clinical features, extra-articular manifestations, differential diagnosis, investigations and management of rheumatoid arthritis (4).	1096	Aug 14
2. Mention the seronegative arthropathies. Describe the clinical features and diagnosis of ankylosing spondylitis.	1104	–
3. Discuss the pathophysiology, clinical features, investigations and management of osteoporosis.	1120	Feb 15
4. Discuss the approach, clinical examination, differential diagnosis and investigations of a comatose patient.	1159	–
5. Discuss the differential diagnosis and investigations of coma in a patient aged 35 years.	1159	–
6. Classify epilepsies. Describe a typical attack of grand mal epilepsy. How do you manage the case of status epilepticus?	1178, 1159	–
7. Classify epilepsy. Discuss the etiopathogenesis and clinical features of epilepsy. Add a note on management of status epilepticus.	1178, 1159	–
8. Classify epilepsy. Discuss their clinical features and management.	1178	–
9. Define seizure and epilepsy. Classify epilepsy. Discuss the clinical features of tonic clonic seizures and its management.	1178	Aug 14

10.	Enumerate the causes of parkinsonism. Describe the approach to management of idiopathic parkinsonism.	1194	Feb 13
11.	Describe the etiology, pathogenesis, clinical features, differential diagnosis and management of parkinsonism (2).	1194	–
12.	Define Parkinson disease and its etiology, clinical features and management.	1194	Feb 15
13.	Discuss the etiopathogenesis, clinical features and management of meningitis.	1201	–
14.	Describe the etiology, clinical features, diagnosis and management of meningococcal meningitis.	1202	–
15.	Discuss the etiology, clinical features, diagnosis and management of pyogenic meningitis.	1202	–
16.	Describe the etiology of meningitis. Elaborate on the clinical features, management and complications of tuberculous meningitis.	1202, 1204	Aug 15
17.	Enumerate the clinical types of central nervous system tuberculosis. Discuss the investigations and treatment of tubercular meningitis.	1204	–
18.	Discuss etiology, clinical features, investigations and management of paraplegia.	1222	–
19.	Mention the causes of peripheral neuropathy. Outline clinical features, investigations and management of acute postinfective polyneuritis.	1223	–
20.	Describe the etiology, pathogenesis, clinical features and management of Guillain-Barré syndrome.	1224	–
21.	Describe etiology, pathology, clinical evaluation and management of myasthenia gravis. Add a note on Lambert-Eaton myasthenic syndrome (LEMS).	1226	–

22.	Define cerebrovascular accident or stroke. Describe the causes, diagnosis and management of cerebral thrombosis.	1234, 1247	–
23.	Discuss the etiopathogenesis and the approach in the management of a patient with cerebrovascular accident.	1234	–
24.	Describe the etiology, clinical features and investigations of cerebral infarction. Describe the role of thrombolytic therapy and angioplasty in cerebral infarction.	1237	–
25.	Define stroke. Discuss pathophysiology, investigations and management of cerebral infarction.	1237	–
26.	Define stroke. Discuss the etiopathogenesis and clinical features of stroke. Outline the management of hemorrhagic stroke.	1237	–
27.	What are the varieties of hemiplegia that you know? Discuss the etiology, clinical features and management of hemorrhagic stroke.	1237	–
28.	Describe the etiology, clinical features, diagnosis and management of ischemic stroke.	1237	–
29.	Mention the causes and management of subarachnoid hemorrhage.	1246	–

SHORT NOTES

1.	Acute gout.	1087	–
2.	Gout (6).	1087	Aug 15
3.	Pseudogout.	1090	–
4.	Rheumatoid arthritis (5).	1096	Feb 12
5.	Disease-modifying antirheumatic drug (DMARD) (2).	1102	–
6.	Seronegative arthritis (3).	1104	–
7.	Reactive arthritis.	1107	Aug 13
8.	Psoriatic arthritis.	1108	Feb 14

9.	Systemic lupus erythematosus (SLE).	1109	Feb 13
10.	SLE classification.	–	–
11.	Raynaud's phenomenon.	1110	–
12.	CREST* syndrome.	1112	–
13.	Polymyositis.	1114	–
14.	Sjögren's syndrome (2).	1114	–
15.	Takayasu's arteritis (2).	1116	Feb 12
16.	Polymyalgia rheumatica.	1117	–
17.	Osteoporosis management.	1122	–
18.	Computed tomography (CT) scan of head.	1149	–
19.	Electroencephalography (EEG).	1151	Feb 13
20.	Lumbar puncture (3).	1153	–
21.	Cerebrospinal fluid (CSF) in meningitis.	1154	–
22.	Phenytoin.	1159, 224, 1184, 1192, 1223	–
23.	Status epilepticus (4).	1159	Aug 12
24.	Brain death.	1160	–
25.	Bell's palsy.	1163	–
26.	Catatonia.	1166	–
27.	Gait.	1168	–
28.	Migraine (3).	1176	Aug 13
29.	Management of migraine.	1177	Feb 12
30.	Trigeminal neuralgia.	1178	–
31.	Febrile seizures.	–	Aug15
32.	Partial seizure.	1179	–
33.	Vestibular neuronitis.	1186	–
34.	Internal ophthalmoplegia.	1190	–
35.	Paraneoplastic syndromes in carcinoma (CA) lung.	1193	Aug 13
36.	Parkinsonism (2).	1194	–
37.	Amyotrophic lateral sclerosis.	1200	–
38.	Bacterial meningitis.	1202	–

*CREST, 'calcinosis, Raynaud's phenomenon, esophageal dysmotility, sclerodactyly and telangiectasia.'

39.	Tuberculous meningitis (3).	1204	–
40.	Antirabies vaccination.	1206	–
41.	Rabies (2).	1206	Feb 12
42.	Rabies prophylaxis.	1206	–
43.	Postexposure prophylaxis of rabies.	1206	Feb 15
44.	Immunization of rabies (2).	1206	–
45.	General paralysis of insane.	1209	–
46.	Tetanus.	1209	–
47.	Tetanus—clinical features (2).	1209	–
48.	Signs and symptoms of increased intracranial tension.	1212	Aug 12
49.	Peripheral neuropathy.	1223	Feb 13
50.	Neuralgic amyotrophy.	1223, 1226	–
51.	Guillain-Barré syndrome.	1224	–
52.	Myasthenia gravis (2).	1226	–
53.	Transient ischemic attack (4).	1239	–
54.	CT in stroke patient.	1241	–
55.	Subtentorial brain tumors.	–	–
56.	Neurosis versus psychosis.	–	–
57.	Circle of Willis.	–	–
58.	Pontine hemorrhage.	–	–
59.	Primitive reflexes.	–	Aug 13
60.	Wasting of small muscles.	–	–
61.	Causes of short stature.	–	–
62.	Claw hand.	–	–
63.	Superficial reflexes.	–	–
64.	Psychomotor epilepsy.	–	–
65.	Brainstem reflexes.	–	–

SHORT ANSWERS

1.	Four causes of polyarthritis.	1069	–
2.	Four causes of proximal muscle weakness.	1077	–
3.	Four clinical features of gout.	1088	Aug 12
4.	Four causes of fever with arthritis.	1094	Feb 13

5. Four extra-articular manifestations of rheumatoid arthritis.	1098	–
6. Four common features of Felty's syndrome.	1100	–
7. Four slow-acting antirheumatic drugs.	1102	–
8. Two drugs used as DMARDs.	1102	–
9. Name any two DMARD.	1102	Feb 14
10. Four types of seronegative spondyloarthritis.	1104	–
11. Four causes of spondyloarthritis.	1104	Feb 12
12. Causes of seronegative arthritis.	1104	–
13. Ankylosing spondylitis.	1105	–
14. Write four extra-articular features of ankylosing spondylitis.	1105	Aug 14
15. Four features of SLE.	1110	–
16. List two diagnostic criteria of SLE.	1111	Aug 15
17. Four features of systemic sclerosis.	1112	Feb 12
18. Henoch-Schönlein purpura.	1119	–
19. Four drugs producing osteoporosis.	1121	–
20. List four causes of Charcot joint.	1133	Feb 12
21. Four causes of carpal tunnel syndrome.	1134	Aug 13
22. List two components of lateral medullary syndrome.	1148	Aug 15
23. List four causes of xanthochromia in CSF analysis.	1154	Feb 12
24. Four complications of lumbar puncture.	1154	Feb 12
25. List any four CSF changes in tuberculous meningitis.	1154	Aug 12
26. Write four secondary causes of headache.	1156	Aug 14
27. List four metabolic causes of coma.	1160	Aug 12
28. Upper motor neuron lesion signs.	1162	Feb 14
29. Bell's palsy (2).	1163	Feb 14
30. List four causes of bilateral facial palsy of LMN type.	1163	Feb 14
31. Catatonia.	1166	–
32. Name four abnormal types of gait.	1168	Feb 14
33. Four gait disorders.	1168	–
34. Horner's syndrome.	1172	–

35.	List two causes of papilledema	1173	Aug 15
36.	Four types of migraine.	1176	Feb 13
37.	List four antiepileptic agents.	1184	Aug 13
38.	Mention four antiepileptic drugs.	1184	–
39.	Name four newer antiepileptic drugs.	1184	Feb 13
40.	List the causes for parkinsonism.	1195	–
41.	Enumerate four clinical features of Parkinson disease.	1195	–
42.	Signs of meningeal irritation (2).	1201	Feb 14
43.	Etiology of pyogenic meningitis.	1202	–
44.	Mention causes of meningitis.	1202	–
45.	List four clinical features of increased intracranial tension.	1212	Feb 12
46.	Four causes of hydrocephalus.	1217	–
47.	Four clinical features of cerebellar disease.	1218	Feb 14
48.	Define TIA* and RIND†.	1239	Feb 14
49.	Four complications of subarachnoid hemorrhage.	1246	Feb 14
50.	Name four neurotransmitters (2).	–	–
51.	List four neurocutaneous syndromes.	–	Aug 14
52.	List four adverse effects of phenytoin.	–	–
53.	List the cranial nerves involved in cavernous sinus thrombosis.	–	Aug 13
54.	List four causes of stroke in young.	–	Feb 15
55.	Prognostic factors in stroke.	–	Feb 13

*TIA, transient ischemic attack; RIND, reversible ischemic neurologic deficit.

Chapter 28

28. Skin Disease

SHORT NOTES

		DVDSN	Recent Years
1.	Staphylococcal scalded skin syndrome (SSSS).	1276	–
2.	Tinea capitis.	1280	–
3.	Scabies (4).	1280	–
4.	Pediculosis.	1281	Feb 12
5.	Seborrheic dermatitis.	1284	–
6.	Psoriasis (6).	1286	Feb 13
7.	Lichen planus.	1289	Aug 13
8.	Urticaria (2).	1290	–
9.	Pemphigus vulgaris.	1293, 1294	–
10.	Hypopigmented skin lesions.	1295	–
11.	Clubbing (3).	1298	–
12.	Skin changes in endocrine diseases.	1299	–
13.	Erythema nodosum.	1303	–
14.	Drug eruptions.	1303	–

SHORT ANSWERS

		DVDSN	Recent Years
1.	Four types of psoriasis.	1286	–
2.	Two causes of diffuse hyperpigmentation.	1296	–

BIBLIOGRAPHY

1. Brain R Walker, Nicki R Colledge, Stuart H Ralston, et al. Davidson's Principles and Practice of Medicine, 22nd edition. Churchill Livingstone Elsevier Limited; 2014.

Section 2

SURGERY

Part I: General Surgery

INSTRUCTIONS TO READERS

- Chapterwise based on MANIPAL MANUAL OF SURGERY, 4th edition (Code: MNPL) with page numbers of answers
- Page numbers of answers from SRB's MANUAL OF SURGERY, 4th edition (Code: SRB) also included
- The year in which questions have recently appeared (last nine question papers from Aug 2011 to Aug 2015) have been mentioned under the recent year's heading
- The number of times a question has been repeated, between 1990 and 2015, is mentioned within brackets along with the respective questions.

Chapters 1 to 8

1. Wound, Keloid, Hypertrophic Scar and Metabolic Response to Injury
2. Acute Infections, Sinus, Fistula and Surgical Site Infection
3. Tetanus and Gas Gangrene
4. Hand and Foot Infections
5. Chronic Infectious Disease
6. Differential Diagnosis of Leg Ulcer and Pressure Sore
7. Lower Limb Ischemia and Popliteal Aneurysm
8. Upper Limb Ischemia and Gangrene

ESSAYS

	MNPL	SRB	Recent Years
1. Discuss the etiology, period of onset, clinical features and management of tetanus.	33	49	–
2. Discuss the etiopathogenesis, clinical features and management of gas gangrene (3).	36	52	Feb 13

3. Classify ulcers. Discuss the pathogenesis, clinical features, investigations and treatment of varicose ulcer secondary to deep vein valve incompetence.	59, 138	15, 249	–
4. Describe the etiopathogenesis, clinical features, differential diagnosis, investigations and management of an early case of Buerger's disease (2).	76	184	–
5. Define thromboangiitis obliterans (Buerger's disease). How will you investigate arterial occlusive disease? Describe the clinical features, complications and management of atherosclerotic gangrene.	76	184, 179, 211	–
6. Describe the etiology, pathogenesis, clinical features, diagnosis and management of thromboangiitis obliterans (TAO) (3).	76	184	–

SHORT NOTES

1. Factors influencing wound healing.	6	7	–
2. Hypertrophic scar (3).	9	12	Aug 12
3. Keloid (2).	9	11	Aug 14
4. Ludwig's angina (2).	16	38, 465	Feb 13
5. Antibioma.	18, 381	42, 558	–
6. Cold abscess.	18	474, 1192	–
7. Hilton's method of draining abscess.	18	43	–
8. Tuberculous lymphadenopathy (3).	19	470	–
9. Tuberculous lymph node.	19	470	–
10. Collar stud abscess.	21	475	–
11. Carbuncle.	23	47	–
12. Necrotizing fasciitis.	24	65	–
13. Tetanus.	33	49	Aug 11
14. Gas gangrene.	36	52	–

15. Paronychia.	41	160	–
16. Deep palmar abscess.	44	162	–
17. Madura foot.	47	57	–
18. Chancre.	54	28, 56	–
19. Gumma.	55	28, 56	–
20. Acquired immunodeficiency syndrome (AIDS) (2).	55	63	–
21. Universal precautions (2).	56	65	Aug 11, Aug 13
22. Ulcer edge.	60, 61	14	–
23. Varicose ulcers (2).	64, 138	28, 249	–
24. Venous ulcer.	64, 138	28, 249	–
25. Trophic ulcer.	65	21, 214	–
26. Bedsore.	72	214	–
27. Buerger's disease (2).	81, 82	184	Aug 15
28. TAO (2).	81, 82	184	Aug 13
29. Color Doppler in peripheral vascular disease.	83	179	–
30. Arterial emboli.	89	197	Aug 11
31. Cervical rib.	101	457	–

SHORT ANSWERS

1. Factors influencing wound healing.	6	7	–
2. Name four differences between keloid and hypertrophic scar.	9	12	–
3. Keloid.	9	11	–
4. Tuberculous lymphadenitis.	19	470	–
5. Collar stud abscess.	21	475	Aug 12, Aug 14
6. Milian's ear sign.	24	39	–
7. Orocutaneous fistula.	28	30	Feb 12
8. Prevention of tetanus.	36	52	Aug 14
9. Paronychia.	41	160	–
10. Acute paronychia.	41	160	Feb 15
11. Ingrowing toenail.	41	172	Aug 12

12.	Universal precaution.	56	65	Aug 11
13.	Ulcer edges.	60, 61	14	Aug 12
14.	Surgery in diabetic patient.	69	213	–
15.	Intermittent claudication (2).	77	175	Feb 13
16.	Dry gangrene.	79	177, 212	Feb 15
17.	Ankle systolic pressure index.	83	180	Aug 11
18.	Arteriogram.	84	180	–
19.	Lumbar sympathectomy.	87	194	Feb 14
20.	Raynaud's disease.	98	189, 216	Feb 14
21.	Adson's test.	102	179, 458	–
22.	Tinel's sign.	–	275	–
23.	Name four differences between exudate and transudate.	–	–	–
24.	Difference between exudate and transudate.	–	–	Aug 12
25.	Mention the branches of external carotid artery.	–	–	–

Chapters 9 to 16

9. Lymphatics, Lymph Vessels and Lymphoma
10. Varicose Veins and Deep Vein Thrombosis
11. Skin Tumors
12. Hemorrhage, Shock and Blood Transfusion
13. Burns, Skin Grafting and Flaps
14. Acid-base Balance, Fluid and Electrolytes
15. Tumors and Soft Tissue Sarcomas
16. Cystic Swellings, Neck swellings and Metastatic Lymph Node Neck

ESSAYS

	MNPL	SRB	Recent Years
1. Discuss the causes of lymphedema. What are the types of lymphedema? Describe the stages and management of filarial lymphedema.	110, 116	257, 259	–
2. Discuss the etiopathology, clinical features, diagnosis and management of varicose veins (2).	127, 130	235	Aug 12
3. Discuss the etiology, types, clinical features, complications and management of varicose veins (2).	127, 130	235	–
4. Discuss the etiology of unilateral swelling of lower limb. What are the various clinical tests you would perform in varicose veins of lower limb? Briefly outline the pathology and management of varicose ulcer.	131, 138	237, 249	–
5. Patient has ulcer near right medial malleolus. How will you evaluate and treat?	138	249	Feb 15
6. Describe the etiopathology, clinical features, diagnostic tests, preventive measures and management of deep vein thrombosis.	140	231	–

7. Discuss the clinical features, diagnosis, clinical staging, investigations and management of malignant melanoma (2).	156	308	-
8. Classify hemorrhage. Discuss briefly the treatment of hemorrhage.	170	121	-
9. Definition and types of shock. Discuss etiology, pathophysiology and management of septic shock.	172	111, 114	-
10. Classify shock. Describe clinical features of shock. Describe investigations and management of septic shock.	172	111, 114	-
11. A 40-year-old man was brought to the hospital with 50% partial thickness burns with deep circumferential burns of right upper limb. Discuss the management and complications.	185	134	-
12. Classify burns. Briefly outline the pathophysiology, immediate resuscitation, complications and management of burn wound.	185	130, 134	-
13. Discuss the pathophysiology of burns. How do you manage a patient with 30% burns? Add a note on postburn sequelae (2).	185	132	-
14. Describe the management and clinical features of secondaries in neck lymph nodes.	263	475	Aug 11

SHORT NOTES

1. Hodgkin's disease.	118	265	-
2. Hodgkin's lymphoma.	118	265	-
3. Modified Perthes' test.	132	239	-
4. Complications of varicose vein.	137	240	Aug 14
5. Varicose ulcer.	138	249	Feb 13
6. Deep vein thrombosis (3).	140	231	Aug 11, Feb 13

7. Marjolin's ulcer (3).	145	13, 24, 28	Aug 13, Feb 14
8. Rodent ulcer (3).	146	24, 303	Aug 12
9. Basal cell carcinoma.	146	24, 303	Feb 15
10. Epithelioma.	151	24, 299	–
11. Squamous cell carcinoma face (2).	151	299	–
12. Squamous cell carcinoma.	151	299	Aug 12
13. Malignant melanoma (2).	156	308	Aug 13
14. Multiple organ dysfunction syndrome (MODS).	171	112, 117	–
15. Septic shock.	173	114	–
16. Cardiac tamponade.	175	1210	–
17. Blood transfusion and its complication.	177, 179	124, 125	Aug 13
18. Complications of transfusion.	179	125	Aug 15
19. Transfusion reactions.	179	125, 126	–
20. Autotransfusion.	180	127	–
21. Volume expanders.	180	126	–
22. Inhalation injury.	186	141	–
23. Burns—fluid therapy.	187	135	Aug 11
24. Split skin graft (3).	189	340	–
25. Metabolic acidosis (3).	196	99	Aug 15
26. Hypokalemia.	204	97	Aug 11
27. Enteral nutrition.	207	102	Feb 15
28. Lipoma (3).	215	71	Aug 12, Feb 12
29. Neurofibroma (2).	218	90	Feb 13
30. Classification of cyst.	232	74	–
31. Dermoid cyst (2).	234	75	–
32. Epidermal cyst.	236	79	–
33. Ganglion.	238	93	Feb 13
34. Baker's cyst (3).	240	87	–
35. Cystic hygroma (3).	241	89, 464	–
36. Ranula (2).	242	389	Feb 14
37. Meningocele.	244	1188	–

38.	Thyroglossal cyst (8).	247	487	Aug 12, Aug 13, Feb 14
39.	Branchial cyst (2).	251	459	–
40.	Branchial fistula.	253	460	–
41.	Carotid body tumor.	254	468	–
42.	Pharyngeal pouch.	256	462	–
43.	Hemangioma.	257	221	–
44.	Arteriovenous fistula.	259	225	–
45.	Cirsoid aneurysm.	262	225	–
46.	Pancoast tumor.	270	1208	–
47.	Lymph cyst (2).	–	88	Aug 12

SHORT ANSWERS

1.	Saphena varix.	130	238, 822	Aug 13
2.	Sclerosing agents.	135	242	–
3.	Varicose vein complications.	137	240	–
4.	Venous ulcer.	64, 138	249	–
5.	Rodent ulcer.	146	24, 303	–
6.	Melanoma.	156	308	–
7.	Reactionary hemorrhage.	170	121	–
8.	Blood transfusion.	177	124	–
9.	Indications for blood transfusion.	177	124	Feb 15
10.	Parkland's formula for burns.	187	135	Aug 13
11.	Split skin graft (SSG).	189	340	Feb 13
12.	Thiersch skin graft.	189	340	–
13.	Flaps.	190	344	Feb 14
14.	Causes of hypercalcemia.	205	532	–
15.	Lipoma.	214	71	–
16.	Dercum disease (2).	215	71	Feb 13
17.	Name four sarcomas, which predominantly spread by lymphatic route.	225	292	–
18.	Kaposi 's sarcoma.	230	328	–
19.	Cystic hygroma (2).	241	89, 464	Aug 15

20.	Lymphangioma.	241	88	Feb 13
21.	Ranula.	242	389	Feb 13
22.	Name four swellings, which give cross-fluctuation.	243	94	–
23.	Thyroglossal cyst.	247	487	–
24.	Hemangioma (2).	257	221	Aug 11, Feb 14
25.	Arteriovenous (AV) fistula.	259	225	–
26.	Branham sign.	262	228	–
27.	False aneurysm.	–	202	–

Chapters 17 to 21

17. Oral Cavity, Odontomes Lip and Palate
18. Salivary Glands
19. Thyroid Gland
20. Parathyroid and Adrenals
21. Breast

ESSAYS

	MNPL	SRB	Recent Years
1. Describe the pathology, clinical features, investigations and management of carcinoma buccal mucosa.	277	396	–
2. Discuss the etiology, pathology and surgical management of carcinoma tongue.	283	417	Feb 14
3. Discuss the differential diagnosis of ulcers of the tongue. Outline the management of early carcinoma tongue.	291, 285	415, 421	–
4. Describe the surgical anatomy of parotid gland and discuss the etiology, clinical features, diagnosis and management of pleomorphic adenoma (2).	302, 307	431, 441	–
5. Classify parotid tumors. How will you evaluate parotid swelling? What are the principles of managing different malignant parotid tumors?	307	440	Aug 15
6. Classify salivary gland tumors. Discuss clinical features, investigations and management of pleomorphic adenoma of parotid gland (2).	307	440, 441	Aug 13
7. Describe the surgical anatomy of thyroid gland. Discuss etiology, clinical features, diagnosis and management of solitary nodule of thyroid.	319, 350	484, 494	–

8.	Classify the swellings of thyroid. Discuss the signs, symptoms, investigations and management of secondary thyrotoxicosis.	326, 331	490, 499	-
9.	Classification of goiter. Discuss the types, etiology, pathology, clinical features, investigations and management of thyrotoxicosis. Add a note on the complications following thyroid surgery (2).	326, 331, 1164	490, 499, 525	-
10.	Describe in detail the clinical features and management of a multinodular goiter.	327	491	Aug 14
11.	Describe the clinical features, investigations and management of thyrotoxicosis (2).	331	499	-
12.	Discuss the clinical features and the management of diffuse toxic goiter.	331	499	-
13.	Discuss the etiopathology, clinical findings, investigations and management of malignancy of thyroid.	338	509	-
14.	Discuss the clinical features and the management of papillary carcinoma of thyroid gland.	338	510	-
15.	Describe in detail the diagnosis and management of a nodule in thyroid.	350	494	Aug 11
16.	Discuss etiology, pathology, clinical features and surgical management of parathyroid adenoma.	363	532	-
17.	Describe the surgical anatomy of the breast. Write the etiology, pathology, clinical features and treatment of fibroadenosis of the breast.	378, 385	544, 551	-
18.	Surgical anatomy of breast. Details about fibroadenoma breast.	378, 388	544, 548	-
19.	Describe the lymphatic drainage of breast. Write about etiology, clinical features and staging of carcinoma breast.	378, 393	546, 563	-

20.	Discuss the benign lesions of the breast and describe the clinical features, pathology and management of carcinoma of breast.	379, 393	548, 563	–
21.	Etiopathogenesis, clinical features and management of carcinoma breast (T2N1M0).	393	563	–
22.	Clinical features and management of carcinoma breast (T2N2M0).	393	563	–
23.	Discuss the etiology, clinical features, pathology, investigations and management of carcinoma of breast (2).	393	563	Aug 12
24.	Discuss the spread of cancer of the breast.	400	569	–
25.	How is breast cancer staged? What is the treatment of stage I and stage II breast cancer?	401, 406	573, 579	Feb 15

SHORT NOTES

1.	Predisposing factors and premalignant conditions in oral cavity malignancy.	273	394	Feb 15
2.	Management of carcinoma tongue.	283	421	–
3.	Tongue tie.	–	417	–
4.	Dental cyst (2).	292	385	–
5.	Adamantinoma (2).	293	383	–
6.	Epulis.	295	382	–
7.	Alveolar abscess.	–	386	–
8.	Parotid abscess.	304	438	–
9.	Submandibular salivary gland.	304	432	Feb 12
10.	Mixed parotid tumor (2).	307	441	Feb 13
11.	Parotid tumors.	307	441	Aug 11
12.	Pleomorphic adenoma.	307	441	Aug 11
13.	Warthin's tumor (2).	311	444	Feb 14
14.	Peripheral nerve injury.	316	273	–
15.	Retrosternal goiter.	331	497	–
16.	Radioactive iodine (2).	337	508	Aug 15

17.	Papillary carcinoma thyroid.	338	510	–
18.	Solitary thyroid nodule (2).	350	494	Aug 14
19.	Hashimoto's thyroiditis (3).	354	519	Aug 15
20.	Riedel's thyroiditis.	355	520	–
21.	Post-thyroidectomy complications (2).	355	524	Feb 13
22.	Thyroid storm.	356	525	Feb 14
23.	Differential diagnosis of hyperparathyroidism.	363	532	–
24.	Parathyroid adenoma.	363	532	–
25.	Conn's syndrome.	369	540	–
26.	Pheochromocytoma.	372	542	–
27.	Acute bacterial mastitis.	379	555	–
28.	Breast abscess (2).	379	556	Feb 13
29.	Cystosarcoma phyllodes (4).	382	552	Aug 14
30.	Mastalgia.	386	553	Feb 15
31.	Fibroadenoma breast (8).	388	548	Aug 11, Aug 12, Aug 14
32.	Nipple retraction.	398	597	–
33.	Fine-needle aspiration cytology (FNAC) (3).	402	289	–

SHORT ANSWERS

1.	Name four premalignant conditions of oral cavity.	273	394	–
2.	Premalignant lesions of oral cavity.	273	394	Aug 12
3.	Leukoplakia.	273	392	–
4.	Submucous fibrosis.	274	393	Aug 15
5.	Differential diagnosis of ulcer tongue.	291	415	–
6.	Dentigerous cyst.	293	384	Feb 14
7.	Adamantinoma (2).	293	383	Feb 13, Aug 15
8.	Tongue tie.	–	417	Aug 12, Aug 14
9.	Danger area of face.	–	–	Feb 12
10.	Frey syndrome (3).	314	452	Feb 13, Aug 14

11.	Exophthalmos.	333	503	Feb 14
12.	Pretibial myxedema (2).	335	504	Aug 13, Feb 15
13.	Antithyroid drugs.	336	506	-
14.	Radioactive iodine.	337	508	Aug 12
15.	Iodine 131.	337	508	-
16.	Lateral aberrant thyroid.	341	489	Aug 13
17.	Multiple endocrine neoplasia (MEN) type II.	348	536	-
18.	Hashimoto's thyroiditis.	354	519	Aug 11
19.	Lingual thyroid (2).	357	486	Feb 12, Aug 12
20.	Trousseaus sign.	362	538	-
21.	Tetany.	362	537	Aug 11
22.	Lymphatic drainage of breast.	378	546	-
23.	Breast abscess.	379	556	-
24.	Antibioma (2).	18, 381	42, 558	Aug 12
25.	Cystosarcoma phyllodes.	382	552	Aug 11
26.	Phyllodes tumor.	382	552	Aug 14
27.	Aberrations of normal development and involution (ANDI) (2).	384	548	Feb 13
28.	Galactocele.	390	554	Feb 14
29.	Gynecomastia.	392	560	-
30.	Triple assessment of breast lump.	400	574	Aug 15
31.	List out four investigations in case of breast lump.	400	574	-
32.	FNAC (2).	402	289	Feb 13
33.	Trucut biopsy.	402	289	Feb 14
34.	QUART* regimen.	407	588	-
35.	QUART.	407	588	Aug 12, Aug 14
36.	Neoadjuvant therapy.	412	755	Aug 11, Aug 14
37.	Mondor's disease.	421	558	-

*QUART—quadrantectomy, axillary dissection and radiotherapy.

Part II: Gastrointestinal Surgery

Chapters 22 to 23

	MNPL	SRB	Recent Years
ESSAYS			
1. Discuss etiology, clinical features, diagnosis and management of carcinoma esophagus.	442	858	–
2. Describe the anatomy, clinical features, investigations and treatment of different types of esophageal atresia and tracheoesophageal fistula.	457	857	–
3. Describe briefly surgical anatomy of stomach. Discuss etiopathology, clinical features, investigations and treatment of carcinoma stomach.	460, 487	869, 902	–
4. Describe the surgical anatomy of stomach. Describe the etiology, pathology, clinical features, diagnosis, investigations and management of benign gastric ulcer.	460, 467	869, 879	–
5. Describe the lymphatic drainage of stomach. Discuss the clinical features, evaluation and management of linitis plastica.	462, 490	871, 908	–
6. Define peptic ulcer. Discuss the etiology, pathogenesis, pathology and management of duodenal ulcer. Add a note on modern advances.	467	882	–

7.	Describe the etiology, clinical features and management of gastric ulcer in a man aged 40 years. Mention the early and late complications that can follow partial gastrectomy.	468, 505	879, 894	–
8.	Enumerate the complications of peptic ulcer disease. Describe the clinical features, diagnosis and treatment of chronic duodenal ulcer.	475, 470	882, 883, 885	–
9.	Discuss the clinical features and the management of perforated duodenal ulcer.	476	887	–
10.	Enumerate the causes of hematemesis. Discuss its management.	480	893	–
11.	What are the causes of hematemesis? How do you manage a case of hematemesis secondary to bleeding peptic ulcer?	480	893, 891	–
12.	Mention causes of acute upper gastrointestinal bleed. How will you investigate and manage a patient of bleeding duodenal ulcer?	480	893, 891	–
13.	Describe in detail the etiopathogenesis, pathology, clinical features, diagnosis, investigations and management of carcinoma stomach (3).	487	902	Aug 13
14.	Describe the surgical anatomy of duodenum. Discuss the clinical features, investigations and management of perforated duodenal ulcer.	512, 476	871, 882	–

SHORT NOTES

1.	Hiatus hernia.	435	847	–
2.	Plummer-Vinson syndrome.	438	853	–
3.	Achalasia cardia (2).	439	850	–
4.	*Helicobacter pylori.*	464	875	–

5. Causes of upper gastrointestinal (UGI) bleed.	480	1061	–
6. Etiology of cancer stomach.	488	902	Feb 15
7. Early gastric cancer.	490	904	Feb 14
8. Postoperative complications of vagotomy.	503	921	Aug 13
9. Postoperative complications of gastrectomy.	505	919	–
10. Duodenal fistula.	506	895	–
11. Congenital pyloric stenosis.	510	876	–
12. Troisier's sign.	–	907	–

SHORT ANSWERS

1. Achalasia cardia.	439	850	Aug 11
2. Stages of peritonitis in duodenal perforation.	476	887	Aug 11
3. Flexible endoscopy.	481	842, 874	Aug 14
4. Hourglass stomach.	487	882	Aug 11
5. Linitis plastica.	490	908	Aug 11, Feb 13
6. Wilke's syndrome.	511	898	Aug 13
7. Troisier's sign.	–	907	Aug 12

Chapters 24 to 26

24. Liver
25. Gall Bladder and Pancreas
26. Spleen

ESSAYS

	MNPL	SRB	Recent Years
1. Describe the surgical anatomy of the liver lobes. Discuss the pathology, clinical features investigations and management of amebic liver abscess.	516, 519	627, 631	–
2. Mention the main functions of liver. What are the routinely available tests for liver function? Discuss the clinical features, diagnosis and management of amebic liver abscess (2).	517, 519	628, 631	–
3. Discuss the clinical features and the management of hydatid disease of the liver.	522	637	–
4. Etiology, pathogenesis, clinical features, complications and management of hydatid cyst of liver.	522	637	–
5. Enumerate the causes of hematemesis. What are the clinical features of portal hypertension? Describe the investigations and management of esophageal variceal bleeding.	480, 537	893, 651, 654	–
6. Describe briefly the surgical anatomy of gallbladder. Discuss the clinical features, investigations and treatment of acute cholecystitis in clinical practice.	550, 556	684, 669	–
7. Describe etiopathogenesis of gallstones, investigations and treatment.	552	679	Feb 15

8.	Etiology, pathology, clinical features and management of calculus cholecystitis.	556	684	–
9.	Discuss the etiology, pathology, clinical features, investigations, complications and treatment of chronic cholecystitis.	560	688	–
10.	Discuss etiology, clinical features and management of obstructive jaundice (2).	564	695	Aug 14
11.	Discuss the etiology, investigations and management of surgical jaundice.	564	695	–
12.	Discuss the etiology of obstructive jaundice. Discuss the clinical features, diagnosis and management of stone in common bile duct.	566	695, 679	–
13.	Describe etiology, pathology, clinical features and management of carcinoma of pancreas.	591, 566	747	Aug 15
14.	Describe tumors of the pancreas. Discuss clinical features, investigations and management of carcinoma head of pancreas.	591, 566	746	–
15.	Discuss the etiology, clinical classification of pancreatitis, investigations and management in brief.	597, 582	727	–
16.	Discuss the etiology, pathology, pathogenesis, clinical features, investigations, management and complications of acute pancreatitis (2).	597	727	Aug 13
17.	Describe the surgical anatomy of spleen. Discuss the etiology, clinical features and management of splenic rupture (2).	617, 619	711, 712	–
18.	Discuss the etiopathology, diagnosis and management of splenic injury.	619	712	–

19. Classify hemorrhage. Discuss the clinical features, management and sequelae of splenic rupture.	170, 619	121, 712	–
20. Enumerate the causes of hemoperitoneum. Discuss the clinical features, diagnosis and management of traumatic rupture of spleen (2).	619	712	–
21. Different causes of splenomegaly. Surgical management of portal hypertension.	628, 542	716, 659	Aug 15

SHORT NOTES

1. Hydatid disease of liver (4).	522	637	–
2. Hydatid cyst of liver.	522	637	Aug 15
3. Hepatitis B.	528	643	–
4. Gallstone.	552	679	Feb 14
5. Biliary stones.	552	679	–
6. Cholelithiasis.	552	679	–
7. Gallstone complications.	554	682	–
8. Mucocele of gallbladder.	561	688	–
9. Stone in common bile duct (CBD).	566	690	–
10. Courvoisier's law.	567	694	–
11. Choledochal cyst (3).	580	675	Feb 13, Feb 15
12. Cholangiocarcinoma.	587	702	–
13. Biliary atresia.	588	677	–
14. APUDoma* (2).	595	536	–
15. Acute pancreatitis.	597	727	–
16. Ranson's criteria.	602	734	Feb 14
17. Pseudopancreatic cyst (6).	607	734	Aug 12, Aug 14
18. Splenic injury.	619	712	–
19. Postsplenectomy complications (3).	623	721	–

*APUD, amine precursor uptake and decarboxylation

20. Tumor markers.	347, 530, 568, 715 977, 997	290, 291	–

SHORT ANSWERS

1. Amebic liver abscess.	519	631	Aug 11
2. Hydatid cyst.	522	637	Aug 11
3. Sites of portosystemic anastomosis.	538	652	Aug 13
4. Esophageal varices.	538	654	Aug 14
5. What is Calot's triangle? What are its contents?	551	670	–
6. Calot's triangle.	551	670	Aug 12, Aug 13, Aug 14
7. Complications of gallstones.	554	682	–
8. Courvoisier's law.	567	694	Aug 12
9. Endoscopic retrograde cholangiopancreatography (ERCP).	569, 584	671	Feb 14
10. Whipple's triad.	596	756	–
11. Annular pancreas.	610	759	Feb 15
12. Indications for splenectomy.	623	720	Aug 13
13. Four causes for splenomegaly.	628	716	–

Chapters 27 to 32

27. Peritoneum, Peritoneal Cavity, Mesentery and Retroperitoneum
28. Small Intestine
29. Large Intestine
30. Intestinal Obstruction
31. Rectum and Anal Canal
32. Lower Gastrointestinal Bleeding

ESSAYS

	MNPL	SRB	Recent Years
1. What are the causes of peritonitis? Describe the clinical features, investigations, complications and management of perforated peptic ulcer.	635, 476	600, 887	–
2. Describe the clinical features and the management of subphrenic abscess.	648	608	–
3. Discuss the etiology, clinical features, pathophysiology, evaluation and management of ileocecal tuberculosis.	673	616	–
4. Etiology, pathology, clinical features and management of acute intestinal obstruction.	729	983	–
5. Discuss the etiology, pathology and surgical management of sigmoid volvulus.	738	997	Feb 14
6. Discuss the differential diagnosis of acute abdomen. How will you reach a diagnosis? Describe the clinical features, investigations and treatment of acute intussusception in a 10-month-old baby.	749	994	–

7. Describe the etiology, pathology, clinical features and diagnosis and management of carcinoma rectum (3).	774	1023	Feb 13, Aug 14
8. Describe the various perianal suppurations and their management.	798	1049	–

SHORT NOTES

1. Peritonitis complications.	647	605	–
2. Meconium peritonitis.	–	993	–
3. Subdiaphragmatic abscess.	648	609	Feb 12
4. Mesenteric cyst.	658	611	Feb 12
5. Retroperitoneal tumors.	661	765	Feb 12
6. Surgical complications of typhoid (2).	686	928	–
7. Peutz-Jeghers syndrome.	689	937, 962	–
8. Carcinoid tumor (5).	692, 837	939	Feb 13, Aug 14
9. Colonoscopy.	707, 1058	1022	–
10. Meckel's diverticulum (3).	741	923	–
11. Gallstone ileus.	747	703	Aug 13
12. Intussusception (5).	749	994	Aug 12, Feb 15
13. Congenital megacolon.	758	949	–
14. Pseudointestinal obstruction.	765	974	–
15. Colostomy.	785	975	Aug 14
16. Prolapse rectum.	787	1030	–
17. Complications of hemorrhoids.	794	1042	–
18. Ischiorectal abscess.	798	1050	Aug 12
19. Fistula in ano (4).	799	1051	Aug 12
20. Pilonidal sinus.	804	1036	–
21. Hidradenitis suppurativa.	809	46, 1060	–
22. Rectal polyp (2).	–	1023	–

SHORT ANSWERS

1.	Foramen of Winslow.	649	609	–
2.	Colonic polyps.	704	961	–
3.	Predisposing factors for sigmoid volvulus.	738	997	–
4.	Meckel's diverticulum.	741	923	Aug 12
5.	Intussusception.	749	994	Feb 14
6.	Treatment of paralytic ileus.	765	1000	–
7.	Temporary colostomy.	785	975	–
8.	Prolapse pile mass.	793	1039	–
9.	Fistula in ano.	799	1051	Aug 11
10.	Anal fissure.	802	1046	Aug 13
11.	Murphy's triad (2).	828	1008	–
12.	Bubonocele.	845	802, 804	–
13.	Lipoma of cord.	849	71, 805	–

Chapters 33 to 37

ESSAYS

	MNPL	SRB	Recent Years
1. Describe the various positions of vermiform appendix. Describe the etiology, pathology, investigations, clinical features and treatment of appendicular lump.	825, 832	1005, 1014	–
2. Discuss briefly about appendicitis. Add etiology, clinical features, investigations and management of appendicular lump.	826, 832	1006	–
3. Discuss briefly the clinical features and the management of acute appendicitis.	826	1006	–
4. Discuss the complications of inguinal hernia. Diagnosis and treatment of strangulated inguinal hernia.	854	817	–
5. Discuss the etiopathogenesis, clinical features, management of obstructed inguinal hernia.	854	817	Feb 14
6. Describe the clinical features and the management of strangulated inguinal hernia.	855	817	–
7. Discuss the etiology, clinical features and management of renal injuries.	896	1080	–
8. Discuss the differential diagnosis (DD) of lump in the right iliac fossa.	909	781	–

9.	Discuss the differential diagnosis of lump in the right iliac fossa. Discuss etiology, clinical features, diagnosis and management of carcinoma cecum.	909, 707	781, 964	-
10.	Discuss the differential diagnosis of painful lump in right iliac fossa in a 20-year-old lady. Describe the clinical features, investigations and management of appendicular lump.	909, 832	781, 1014	-

SHORT NOTES

1.	Management of appendicular mass (2).	833	1015	Aug 13
2.	Appendicular abscess (3).	834	1015	Aug 14
3.	Obstructed femoral hernia.	860	822	-
4.	Femoral hernia (4).	860	822	Aug 13
5.	Umbilical hernia.	863	829	-
6.	Incisional hernia (2).	866	825	Aug 14
7.	Epigastric hernia.	870	831	-
8.	Fatty hernia of linea alba.	870	831	-
9.	Spigelian hernia.	871	833	-
10.	Desmoid tumor (2).	882	791	-
11.	Blast injuries.	898	147	-

SHORT ANSWERS

1.	Pilonidal sinus.	804	1036	Aug 12, Aug 14
2.	Complications of perforated appendix.	834	1007	-
3.	Surgical anatomy of inguinal canal.	842	800	-
4.	Strangulated hernia.	855	817	Aug 14
5.	Richter hernia (2).	858	834	Feb 13

6.	Umbilical hernia.	863	829	Feb 13
7.	Epigastric hernia.	870	831	Feb 14
8.	Spigelian hernia.	871	833	Aug 12
9.	Umbilical granuloma.	878	786	Feb 12
10.	Desmoid tumor (3).	882	791	Aug 12, Feb 14

Part III: Urology

Chapters 38 to 43

	MNPL	SRB	Recent Years
ESSAYS			
1. Discuss the surgical anatomy of kidney. Write about the etiology, clinical features and treatment of renal tuberculosis.	932, 943	1065, 1081	–
2. Discuss the etiology, varieties and clinical features of renal calculus. Give a brief account on the investigations and treatment of a calculus in the renal pelvis.	935	1089	–
3. Enumerate etiopathology and clinical features of renal stones. Discuss recent trends in management of urolithiasis.	935	1089	–
4. Describe the etiology, clinical features and management of hydronephrosis.	939	1084	–
5. Discuss the causes, clinical features, investigations and management of hydronephrosis in children.	939	1084	–
6. Describe the causes, clinical features, investigations and treatment of a case of unilateral hydronephrosis of kidney (2).	939	1084	–

7. Write the etiology and management of bilateral hydronephrosis (2).	940	1084	-
8. Discuss pathology, clinical features and management of Wilms' tumor (2).	946	1099	Aug 12
9. Discuss the causes of hematuria. How do you diagnose, investigate and manage Wilms' tumor?	1002, 946	1075, 1099	-
10. Describe causes of hematuria. Discuss etiopathogenesis, clinical features and management of hypernephroma.	1002, 947	1075, 1100	-
11. Classify neoplasms of the kidney. Discuss the clinical features, etiopathology, diagnosis and management of hypernephroma (2).	945, 947	1098, 1100	-
12. What are the types of rupture of urinary bladder? Describe the clinical features, diagnosis and management.	962	1115	-
13. What are the causes of acute retention of urine? Describe the clinical features, investigations and treatment of benign enlargement of prostate (2).	968, 973	1136, 1122	-
14. Discuss the etiology, pathology, clinical features, investigations, medical and surgical management of benign enlargement of prostate.	973	1122	-
15. Describe in detail the etiology, pathology, clinical features and surgical management of carcinoma penis (3).	982	1142	Aug 11, Feb 13
16. Discuss the etiology, clinical features and management of undescended testis.	992	1161	-

17.	Classify testicular tumors. Discuss clinical features, investigations and management of the same.	994	1166	–
18.	Classification of testicular tumors. Discuss the clinical features, investigations, diagnosis and management of seminoma testis (2).	994	1166	–
19.	Classify testicular tumor. Discuss the etiopathology, clinical features, investigations and management of teratoma (2).	994	1166	Feb 12
20.	How do you classify testicular tumors? Discuss the pathology, clinical features and management of seminoma and teratoma.	994	1166	–
21.	Describe the various causes for scrotal swelling. Describe the clinical features and management of seminoma testis.	991, 995	1166	–
22.	Discuss the differential diagnosis of hematuria in a geriatric patient.	1002	1075	–

SHORT NOTES

1.	Intravenous pyelography.	924	1067	–
2.	Renal calculus.	935	1089	–
3.	Dietl's crisis.	941	1084, 1086	–
4.	Renal tuberculosis.	943	1081	Aug 13
5.	Wilms' tumor (2).	946	1099	–
6.	Hypernephroma (2).	947	1100	–
7.	Vesical calculus (2).	955	1106	Feb 13
8.	Ectopia vesicae (2).	959	1106	Aug 15
9.	Diverticula of bladder.	960	1118	–
10.	Rupture of urethra.	963	1129	–
11.	Urethral injury.	963	1129	Feb 15
12.	Hypospadias.	967	1132	–
13.	Causes of retention of urine.	968	1136	–

14.	Carcinoma prostate.	975	1126	–
15.	Prostate-specific antigen (PSA).	977	1121	–
16.	Phimosis (4).	981	1138	Feb 13
17.	Etiology of carcinoma (CA) penis.	982	1142	–
18.	Peyronie's disease.	987	1141	–
19.	Lymphogranuloma venereum.	987	29	–
20.	Congenital hydrocele (2).	988	1149	–
21.	Spermatocele.	992	1156	–
22.	Undescended testis (2).	992	1161	Feb 13
23.	Varicocele.	993	1157	–
24.	Ectopic testis.	993	1163	–
25.	Torsion testis (3).	994	1164	Aug 12, Aug 14
26.	Seminoma testis (2).	995	1166	–
27.	Teratoma testis.	995	1166	Feb 14
28.	Hematuria.	1002	1075	–

SHORT ANSWERS

1.	Polycystic kidney.	933	1077	Aug 15
2.	Horseshoe kidney.	935	1076	–
3.	Staghorn calculi.	936	1097	Aug 12
4.	Extracorporeal shock wave lithotripsy (ESWL).	938	1092	–
5.	Wilms' tumor.	946	1099	Aug 11, Feb 14
6.	Indications for urinary diversion.	961	1119	–
7.	Phimosis (2).	981	1138	Aug 13
8.	Paraphimosis.	982	1139	–
9.	Name four premalignant conditions of penile swelling.	982	1142	–
10.	Peyronie's disease.	987	1141	Aug 13
11.	Complications of hydrocele.	991	1152	Aug 13
12.	Complications of pyocele.	991	1155	Aug 14
13.	Spermatocele.	992	1156	Feb 15
14.	Epididymal cyst.	992	1155	–

15.	Torsion of testis (2).	994	1164	Aug 11
16.	Seminoma.	995	1166	–
17.	Tumor markers in testicular tumors.	997	1168	Feb 15
18.	Hematuria.	1002	1075	Feb 14
19.	Anuria.	–	–	Aug 15
20.	Orchitis.	–	1170	–

Part IV and V

Chapters 44 to 53

44. Chest Trauma and Cardiothoracic Surgery
45. Neurosurgery
46. Principles of Radiology
47. Principles of Clinical Radiation Oncology
48. Principles of Anesthesiology (dealt separately at the end)
49. Organ Transplantation
50. X-rays and Images
51. Instruments
52. Specimens
53. Operative Surgery, Laparoscopic Surgery and Accessories

	MNPL	SRB	Recent Years
ESSAYS			
1. Write an essay on organ transplantation.	1108	353	–
SHORT NOTES			
1. Open chest injuries.	1009	1194	Feb 14
2. Flail chest (4).	1010	1196	Feb 13
3. Pneumothorax (3).	1011	1197	Aug 12, Aug 15
4. Tension pneumothorax.	1012	1197	–
5. Patent ductus arteriosus (PDA).	1027	1217	–
6. Coarctation of aorta.	1028	1218	–
7. Lucid interval.	1037	1177	–
8. Acute extradural hematoma (2).	1037	1177	–
9. Glasgow coma scale (2).	1038	1175	Aug 13
10. Hutchinson's pupil.	1038	1177	–
11. Acute subdural hematoma (2).	1039	1178	–
12. Astrocytoma.	1042	1183	–
13. Barium meal series.	1048	873	–

14.	Barium enema.	1049	981	–
15.	Computerized tomography.	1052	1240	–
16.	Ultrasonography.	1052	1238	–
17.	Magnetic resonance imaging (MRI).	1053	1242	–
18.	Berry's aneurysm.	–	1182	–
19.	Types of suture material (2).	1140	1256	Aug 13
20.	Sengstaken tube.	1140	657	Feb 14
21.	Postoperative care for abdominal surgery.	1151	1234	Aug 11
22.	Disinfection.	1152	1244	–
23.	Circumcision (2).	1158	1140	Aug 14
24.	Vasectomy.	1160	1260	–
25.	Tracheostomy.	1161	1263	Aug 13
26.	Colectomy.	1172	958, 971	–
27.	Laparoscopy.	1174	1267	–
28.	Crush syndrome.	–	10	–
29.	Methicillin-resistant *Staphylococcus aureus* (MRSA).	–	–	–
30.	Rhesus (Rh) incompatibility.	–	–	–
31.	Day care surgery.	–	1274	Aug 13

SHORT ANSWERS

1.	Flail chest.	1010	1196	Aug 11, Aug 14
2.	Stove-in-chest.	1011	1196	Aug 15
3.	Pneumothorax.	1011	1197	–
4.	Empyema thoracis.	1018	1199	–
5.	Lucid interval.	1037	1177	–
6.	Glasgow coma scale (2).	1038	1175	–
7.	MRI.	1053	1242	Aug 11, Feb 13
8.	Radioresponsive tumors.	1065	1225	Aug 11
9.	Human leukocyte antigen (HLA) matching.	1108	353	Feb 15
10.	Ryles' tube.	1139	1254	–

11.	Foley catheterization.	1139	1072	Aug 14
12.	Postoperative complications of thyroidectomy.	1164	1263	–
13.	Laparoscopic surgery.	1174	1267	Aug 11
14.	Name four indications for using Romo Vac suction drain.	–	1253	–
15.	Radioisotopes in diagnosis of surgical conditions.	–	1243	–
16.	Pyothorax.	–	–	–
17.	Excision biopsy.	–	289	–
18.	Day care surgery (2).	–	1274	Aug 12

Principles of Anesthesiology

	MNPL	SRB	Recent Years
SHORT NOTES			
1. Preparation of patient for general anesthesia.	1071	1231	–
2. Preanesthetic assessment (2).	1072	1231	–
3. General endotracheal anesthesia.	1074	1232	–
4. General anesthesia.	1074	1232	Feb 15
5. Halothane.	1074	1232	–
6. Nitrous oxide.	1076	1232	–
7. Thiopentone sodium.	1076	1232	–
8. Intravenous anesthesia (2).	1076	1235	–
9. Pancuronium bromide.	1079	1232	–
10. Muscle relaxants (6).	1079	1232	–
11. Succinylcholine.	1079	1232	Feb 14
12. Management of airway in an unconscious patient.	1080	1233	–
13. Neostigmine.	1080	1232	–
14. Endotracheal anesthesia.	1080	1233	Feb 13
15. Endotracheal intubation.	1080	1233	–
16. Endotracheal tube (2).	1082	1233	–
17. Pulse oximeter.	1085	–	–
18. Local anesthesia (3).	1089	1235	–
19. Classification of local anesthetics.	1089	1235	–
20. Local anesthetics (2).	1089	1235	–
21. Common local anesthetic techniques.	1089	1235	–
22. Regional anesthesia (3).	1089	1235	Aug 15
23. Lidocaine.	1089	1235	–
24. Lignocaine toxicity.	1090	1235	–
25. Spinal anesthesia (7).	1091	1235	Aug 12, Aug 14

26.	Postspinal anesthesia headache.	1092	1236	–
27.	Complications of spinal anesthesia (3).	1092	1236	–
28.	Epidural anesthesia (9).	1093	1236	Aug 11
29.	Stages of ether anesthesia.	–	–	–
30.	Stages of general anesthesia.	–	–	–
31.	Field block anesthesia.	1095	1235	–
32.	Nerve block (3).	1095	1235	Aug 12
33.	Brachial block.	1095	–	–
34.	Ankle block.	1096	1235	–
35.	Postoperative complications of general anesthesia (GA).	1098	1234	–
36.	Cardiopulmonary resuscitation (CPR) (2).	1100	–	–
37.	Cardiac arrest.	1100	–	–
38.	Mouth-to-mouth respiration.	1102	–	–
39.	Boyle's apparatus.	–	1233	Aug 11
40.	Digital block anesthesia.	–	1235	Aug 11
41.	Lumbar puncture.	–	1180	Aug 11

SHORT ANSWERS

1.	Muscle relaxants.	1079	1232	Aug 15
2.	Bupivacaine (2).	1089	1235	Feb 13
3.	Sensorcaine.	–	–	Feb 14
4.	Common local anesthetic techniques.	1089	1235	–
5.	Epidural anesthesia.	1093	1236	Aug 13
6.	Oxygen therapy.	–	1232	–
7.	Ventilators in intensive care unit (ICU).	–	–	–

BIBLIOGRAPHY

1. Rajgopal Shenoy K, Anitha Shenoy. Manipal Manual of Surgery, 4th edition. New Delhi: CBS Publishers and Distributors Pvt Ltd; 2014.
2. Sriram Bhat M. SRB's Manual of Surgery, 4th edition. New Delhi: Jaypee Brothers Medical Publishers (P) Ltd; 2013.

Section 3

ORTHOPEDICS

Orthopedics

INSTRUCTIONS TO READERS

- Chapterwise based on J Maheshwari's ESSENTIAL ORTHOPAEDICS, 5th edition (Code: MHSWRI) with page numbers of answers
- Page numbers of answers from 4th edition is also included within brackets next to it
- Page numbers of answers from Natarajan's TEXTBOOK OF ORTHOPAEDICS AND TRAUMATOLOGY, 7th edition (Code: NTRJN) also included
- The year in which questions have recently appeared (last nine question papers from Aug 2011 to Aug 2015) have been mentioned under the recent year's heading
- The number of times a question has been repeated, between 1990 and 2015, is mentioned within brackets along with the respective questions.

Chapters 1 to 6

1. Orthopedic Trauma: Introduction
2. Anatomy of Bone and Fracture Healing
3. Treatment of Fractures: General Principles
4. Splint and Tractions
5. Recent Advances in the Treatment of Fractures
6. Approach to a Patient with Limb Injury

SHORT NOTES

	MHSWRI	NTRJN	Recent Years
1. Compound fracture.	1 (1)	307	Aug 14
2. Classification of compound fracture.	–	307	–
3. Plaster of Paris.	17 (17)	205	–
4. Thomas splint (2).	25 (24)	260	–
5. Intramedullary fixation of fracture.	30 (29)	262	–

6. Uses of external fixation.	33 (32)	298	Aug 12
7. Bone cement.	–	94	–

SHORT ANSWERS

1. Pathological fracture.	–	202	–
2. Plaster of Paris.	17 (17)	205	–
3. Use of plaster of Paris in orthopedics.	17 (17)	205	Feb 14
4. Ilizarov fixator.	33 (32)	190	Aug 14

Chapters 7 to 12

	MHSWRI	NTRJN	Recent Years
ESSAYS			
1. What are the common deformities of the knee region seen in children and adolescents? Describe their etiology and outline the management.	75 (72)	–	–
SHORT NOTES			
1. Clinical features and diagnosis of fat embolism following fracture shaft of femur.	43 (42)	209	Feb 13
2. Clinical features of acute compartment syndrome.	47 (46)	270	Aug 13
3. Nonunion (3).	48 (47)	210	–
4. Malunion (2).	49 (48)	211	–
5. Myositis ossificans (2).	52 (51)	209	–
6. Nerve injuries.	62 (59)	320	–
7. Saturday night palsy.	– (–)	327	–
8. Foot drop (4).	63 (60)	145	–
9. Wrist drop (3).	63 (60)	323	–
10. Claw hand (4).	64 (61)	147	–
11. Ulnar claw hand (2).	64 (61)	148	Feb 12, Aug 15
12. Erb's palsy.	– (–)	326	–
13. Radial nerve injuries.	65 (62)	323	–
14. Clinical features of radial nerve injury.	65 (62)	323	Feb 13

15.	Clinical features of ulnar nerve palsy.	67 (64)	325	Aug 13
16.	Electromyography.	69 (66)	–	–
17.	Tinel's sign.	69 (66)	322	–
18.	Arthroplasty.	84 (81)	186	–
19.	Bone graft (3).	84 (81)	194	–

SHORT ANSWERS

1.	Nonunion.	48 (47)	210	–
2.	Treatment of hypertrophic nonunion.	48 (47)	210	Aug 12
3.	Malunion.	49 (48)	211	Feb 12
4.	Greenstick fracture.	59 (57)	236	Feb 14
5.	Neurapraxia.	63 (60)	320	–
6.	Ape thumb deformity.	64 (61)	324	–
7.	Erb's palsy (policeman tip deformity).	64 (61)	326	–
8.	Claw hand.	64 (61)	147	Aug 12
9.	Foot drop.	69 (66)	145	Feb 14
10.	Ulnar paradox.	– (–)	–	–

Chapters 13 to 21

13. Injuries Around the Shoulder, Fracture of Humerus
14. Injuries Around the Elbow
15. Injuries of Forearm and Wrist
16. Hand Injuries
17. Pelvic Fractures
18. Injuries Around the Hip
19. Fracture Shaft of Femur
20. Injuries Around the Knee
21. Injuries to Leg, Ankle and Foot

ESSAYS

	MHSWRI	NTRJN	Recent Years
1. A 40-year-old man fell down from the roof hitting back of his neck against the sun shade and landed down on feet over the ground and sustained multiple injuries. Discuss the injuries and their management.	36 (35)	–	–
2. Discuss the classification, clinical features, complications and management of dislocation of shoulder.	89 (86)	218	–
3. Discuss the dislocation of shoulder joint and its management, with special reference to the operative procedures for recurrent dislocation.	89 (86)	218	–
4. Describe etiopathology and clinical features of anterior dislocation of the shoulder. Describe the surgical options in a 20-year-old athlete with recurrent dislocation of shoulder.	89 (86)	218, 220	Aug 12
5. Describe various injuries around elbow joint. Discuss in detail the types, mechanism, clinical features, radiological features, diagnosis, management and complications of supracondylar fracture of humerus (2).	97 (93)	226	–

6.	Enumerate the fractures and dislocations caused by a fall on outstretched hand. Describe the clinical features, complications and management of supracondylar fracture of humerus in a child.	97 (93)	226	–
7.	Describe mechanism of injury, clinical features, complications and management of supracondylar fracture of the humerus in children.	97 (93)	226	Feb 13
8.	Describe the etiology, pathogenesis, pathology, clinical features, investigations, management and complications of supracondylar fracture of humerus (2).	97 (93)	226	–
9.	Classify the type of epiphyseal injuries. Describe the etiology, clinical signs and symptoms, complications and management of fracture of medial condyle of humerus in an 8-year-old child.	–, 105 (–, 101)	212, 229	–
10.	Classify fractures around elbow. Write the X-ray findings, clinical features and management of Colles' fracture and complications.	97, 111 (93,107)	226, 238	–
11.	What are the fractures caused by fall on an outstretched hand? Describe the anatomy, pathology, clinical features, treatment and complications of Colles' fracture (2).	97, 111 (93,107)	238	–
12.	Describe mechanism of injury, clinical features, complications and management of Colles' fracture.	111 (107)	238	Aug 13
13.	Classify traumatic dislocations of the hip. Describe this mode of injury. Outline the principles of management of each type.	130 (126)	250	–

14.	Discuss the classification, clinical features, complications and management of dislocation of hip.	130 (126)	250	-
15.	Discuss the causes of dislocation of hip. Discuss the mechanism, signs and symptoms, diagnosis and treatment of posterior dislocation of hip.	130 (126)	250	-
16.	Classify hip dislocations. Describe the mechanism of injury, symptoms, signs and treatment of traumatic posterior dislocation of hip joint. Add a note on its complication.	130 (126)	251	-
17.	Describe the surgical anatomy of femur. Discuss the clinical features, investigations and management of fracture neck of femur.	129, 132 (125,128)	250, 254	-
18.	Describe the clinical features and management of fracture neck of femur.	132 (128)	254	Aug 11
19.	Describe the anatomy, pathology, classification, clinical features and management of fracture neck of femur (2).	132 (128)	254	-
20.	Classify fracture neck of femur. Mention the blood supply to the head of femur. Describe in detail the treatment of the fracture neck of femur in an adult.	132 (128)	254	-
21.	Classify fracture neck of femur. Describe clinical features, differential diagnosis and management of fracture neck of femur in postmenopausal woman.	132 (128)	254	-
22.	Describe the etiology, clinical features, management and complications of intracapsular fractures of the neck of femur.	132 (128)	254	-

23.	Discuss the etiology, mechanism, clinical features of fracture neck of femur of 60 year individual.	132 (128)	254	–
24.	Describe the mechanism of injury, clinical features, complications and management of fracture neck of femur (intracapsular) in a 70-year-old man.	132 (128)	254	Feb 14
25.	Discuss the pathophysiology, clinical features, investigations and management of trochanteric fracture of femur.	138 (134)	257	–
26.	Describe in detail about intertrochanteric fractures of femur and its management.	138 (134)	256	Feb 12
27.	What is a pathological fracture? Outline briefly how you will investigate and manage an elderly patient admitted with a pathological fracture of shaft of femur (2).	141 (136)	259	–
28.	Discuss the mechanism, classification and management of ankle fractures.	160 (154)	273	–

SHORT NOTES

1.	Clavicle fracture.	88 (85)	215	–
2.	Shoulder dislocation (2).	89 (86)	218	–
3.	Anterior dislocation of shoulder.	89 (86)	218	Aug 15
4.	Recurrent dislocation of shoulder.	89 (86)	220	Aug 14
5.	Kocher's maneuver.	91 (88)	219	–
6.	Supracondylar fracture of humerus (2).	97 (93)	226	–
7.	Volkmann's contracture (3).	102 (98)	207	–
8.	Cubitus varus.	102 (98)	228	Feb 15
9.	Tardy ulnar palsy.	104 (100)	159, 325	–
10.	Monteggia fracture.	110 (106)	236	–
11.	Clinical features and management of Monteggia fracture dislocation.	110 (106)	236	Feb 14
12.	Colles' fracture (5).	111 (107)	238	Feb 12

13. Smith's fracture.	114 (110)	240	–
14. Bennett's fracture.	117 (113)	244	–
15. Mechanism of injury and clinical features of posterior dislocation of hip.	130 (126)	251	Aug 12
16. Fracture of patella (2).	147 (142)	265	–
17. Hemarthrosis.	149 (144)	105	–
18. Management principles of open fracture of the midshaft of tibia with soft tissue loss.	156 (150)	307	Feb 13
19. Pott's fracture.	159 (153)	273	–
20. Fracture of talus.	165 (159)	277	Aug 14
21. Ruptured Achillis tendon.	– (–)	318	–
22. Epiphyseal injury.	– (–)	212	Feb 12
23. Classify epiphyseal injury.	– (–)	212	Aug 12

SHORT ANSWERS

1. Shoulder dislocation.	89 (86)	218	Feb 12
2. Name the nerves injured in the following situations: a. Fracture shaft of humerus. b. Supracondylar fracture.	93, 98 (90, 94)	223, 228	–
3. Volkmann's ischemic contracture.	102 (98)	207	–
4. Tardy ulnar palsy.	104 (100)	159, 325	–
5. Write the typical deformities in: a. Colles' fracture. b. Monteggia fracture.	112, 110 (108, 106)	238, 236	–
6. Mallet finger.	118 (114)	248	Aug 14
7. Write the typical deformities in: a. Posterior dislocation of hip. b. Anterior dislocation of hip.	130, 131 (126,127)	251, 252	–
8. Hemarthrosis.	149 (144)	105	–
9. Ankle joint.	159 (153)	273	Feb 12
10. Differences between quadriceps contusion and quadriceps rupture.	– (–)	317, 267	–

Chapters 22 to 24

22. Infections of Bones and Joints
23. Tuberculosis of Bones and Joints
24. Infections of the Hand

ESSAYS

	MHSWRI	NTRJN	Recent Years
1. Define and classify osteomyelitis. Describe pathogenesis, clinical features, complications and management of chronic non-specific osteomyelitis.	168, 171 (162, 165)	35, 37	–
2. Discuss the etiology, pathology, clinical features and management of acute hematogenous osteomyelitis of lower end of femur and outline its differential diagnosis and complications.	168 (162)	35	–
3. Write briefly about the etiopathology of acute osteomyelitis. Discuss its complications and management in a child.	168 (162)	35	–
4. Describe the pathogenesis, clinical features, complications and management of Pott's spine involving dorsolumbar spine.	185 (179)	53	–
5. Describe in detail the stages, clinical features, investigations and management of tuberculosis of hip joint.	194 (188)	61	–

SHORT NOTES

	MHSWRI	NTRJN	Recent Years
1. Osteomyelitis of humerus (2).	168 (162)	35	–
2. Clinical features and diagnosis of acute osteomyelitis.	168 (162)	35	Aug 12

3.	Clinical features and management of acute osteomyelitis of the tibia in a 7-year-old child.	168 (162)	35	Feb 14
4.	Osteomyelitis (3).	168 (162)	35	Feb 12
5.	Chronic osteomyelitis of tibia (3).	171 (165)	37	–
6.	Sequestrum (3).	172 (166)	38	–
7.	Brodie's abscess.	175 (169)	40	–
8.	Septic arthritis (2).	175 (169)	45	Feb 15
9.	Madura foot.	178 (172)	42	–
10.	Tuberculosis arthritis.	182 (176)	64	–
11.	Tuberculous synovitis.	182 (176)	63	–
12.	Ankylosis.	183 (177)	66	–
13.	Pott's spine.	185 (179)	53	–
14.	Cold abscess (2).	187 (181)	55	–
15.	Psoas abscess.	190 (183)	67	–
16.	Complication of tuberculous spine.	191 (185)	55	Feb 12
17.	Tuberculosis of knee.	199 (193)	67	–
18.	Tuberculous dactylitis.	203 (197)	70	–
19.	Deep palmar abscess.	208 (201)	162	Feb 14

SHORT ANSWERS

1.	Differential diagnosis of acute osteomyelitis.	170 (164)	36	Aug 13
2.	What is sequestrum?	172 (166)	38	Aug 12
3.	Brodie's abscess.	175 (169)	40	Feb 14
4.	Septic arthritis.	175 (169)	45	–
5.	Clinical features of synovitis of the knee joint.	175 (169)	45	Feb 13
6.	Ankylosis.	183 (177)	66	–
7.	Pott's disease of spine.	185 (179)	53	–
8.	Gibbus deformity.	187 (182)	55	Aug 13
9.	Web space infection of hand.	207 (200)	161	–

Chapters 25 to 27

25. Congenital Talipes Equinovarus
26. Congenital Dislocation of the Hip and Other Malformations
27. Poliomyelitis and Other Neuromuscular Disorders

	MHSWRI	NTRJN	Recent Years
SHORT NOTES			
1. Congenital talipes equinovarus (CTEV) (4).	210 (203)	9	–
2. Clinical features and management of clubfoot (congenital talipes equinovarus) (3).	212 (205)	11	Feb 14
3. Surgical treatment of CTEV in a 1-year-old child.	214 (207)	12	Aug 12
4. Management of CTEV.	214 (207)	12	Aug 13
5. Congenital dislocation of hip (3).	219 (212)	13	Feb 13
6. Acute poliomyelitis.	226 (219)	141	–
7. Spina bifida.	230 (223)	22	–
8. Meningomyelocele.	231 (224)	22	–
SHORT ANSWERS			
1. Deformities in a talipes equinovarus and talipes equinovalgus.	211, – (204, –)	9, –	–
2. Define: a. Spondylolysis. b. Spondylolisthesis.	224, 225 (217, 218)	170	–
3. Galeazzi sign.	221 (214)	15	–
4. Ortolani's test.	221 (214)	15	–
5. Ortolani's sign.	221 (214)	15	Aug 13

Chapter 28

28. Bone Tumors

ESSAYS

	MHSWRI	NTRJN	Recent Years
1. Classify the bone tumors. Discuss in detail about the clinical features, investigations and management of Ewing sarcoma (2).	236, 243 (229, 236)	115, 131	-
2. Classify bone tumors. Discuss in details about the clinical features, investigations and management of osteoclastoma (giant cell tumor).	236, 237 (229, 230)	115, 126	-
3. Discuss the classification of bone tumors. Elaborate on the clinical features, investigations and management of osteosarcoma (2).	236, 239 (229, 232)	115, 122	Aug 15
4. Discuss the pathology, clinical features and differential diagnosis of osteosarcoma. How will you treat a case of osteosarcoma of the upper tibia in a 16-year-old boy?	239 (232)	122	-
5. Describe the clinical features and management of osteogenic sarcoma of lower end of femur. Add a note on chemotherapy and radiotherapy.	239 (232)	122	-
6. Classify the usual tumors occurring in the bone. Describe the clinical features, investigations and treatment of osteogenic sarcoma.			

	What are the radiological differences between osteosarcoma and osteoclastoma?	236, 239, 244 (229, 232, 237)	115, 122, 126	-

SHORT NOTES

1.	Osteoid osteoma (4).	235 (228)	118	Aug 12, Aug 14
2.	Osteoclastoma (4).	237 (230)	126	-
3.	Diagnosis of giant cell tumor of proximal tibia.	237 (230)	126	Aug 13
4.	Osteosarcoma (4).	239 (232)	122	Feb 12, Feb 14
5.	Principles of management of established osteosarcoma of distal femur.	240 (233)	122	Feb 13
6.	Codman's triangle.	240 (233)	123	-
7.	Ewing's sarcoma (2).	243 (236)	131	-
8.	Clinical features and management of Ewing's tumor.	243 (236)	131	Feb 14
9.	Chondrosarcoma.	246 (239)	129	-
10.	Metastatic bone disease (2).	246 (239)	134	-
11.	Osteochondroma.	247 (240)	120	-
12.	Bone cyst.	248 (241)	121	-

SHORT ANSWERS

1.	Clinical features of giant cell tumor.	237 (230)	126	Aug 12
2.	X-ray appearance in osteosarcoma.	240 (233)	122	Aug 12
3.	Microscopic pathology of Ewing's sarcoma.	243 (236)	131	Feb 13
4.	Treatment of chondrosarcoma of the proximal femur.	246 (239)	129	Feb 13
5.	Bone secondaries.	246 (239)	134	-
6.	Osteochondroma.	247 (240)	120	Feb 14
7.	X-ray appearance of simple bone cyst.	248 (241)	121	Feb 13

Chapters 29 to 33

29. Prolapsed Intervertebral Disk
30. Approach to a Patient with Back Pain
31. Spinal Injuries
32. Traumatic Paraplegia
33. Scoliosis and Other Spinal Deformities

	MHSWRI	NTRJN	Recent Years
ESSAYS			
1. Describe the complications of traumatic paraplegia. Describe their management.	276 (268)	286	-
SHORT NOTES			
1. Lumbar disk prolapse.	252 (244)	172	-
2. Spondylolisthesis.	283 (275)	170	-

Chapters 34 and 35

34. Arthritis and Related Diseases
35. Degenerative Disorders

	MHSWRI	NTRJN	Recent Years
ESSAYS			
1. Describe the clinical features, manifestations and complications of rheumatoid arthritis.	286 (278)	89	–
SHORT NOTES			
1. Gout.	293 (285)	102	Feb 15
2. Rheumatoid arthritis.	286 (278)	89	Aug 14
3. Neuropathic joint (2).	294 (286)	101	Aug 15
SHORT ANSWERS			
1. Synovial membrane.	– (–)	–	Feb 12
2. Cervical collar.	272 (264)	154	Aug 15
3. Neuropathic joint.	294 (286)	101	–

Chapters 36 to 42

36. Affections of the Soft Tissues
37. Metabolic Bone Diseases
38. Miscellaneous Affections of the Bone
39. Miscellaneous Regional Diseases
40. Amputations, Prosthetics and Orthotics
41. Arthroscopic Surgery
42. Joint Replacement Therapy

	MHSWRI	NTRJN	Recent Years
ESSAYS			
1. Describe the etiology, clinical features and radiological findings of Perthes' disease. Mention the differential diagnosis.	318 (308)	111	–
2. Discuss the etiology, pathological anatomy and clinical features of genu valgum in a 13-year-old girl. Add a note on the management.	324 (314)	177	Feb 15
SHORT NOTES			
1. Tennis elbow (2).	302 (293)	158	–
2. Golfer's elbow.	302 (293)	–	–
3. Trigger finger.	303 (294)	163	–
4. Ganglion (2).	303 (294)	162	–
5. Carpal tunnel syndrome.	303 (294)	163	–
6. Frozen shoulder.	304 (295)	157	–
7. Plantar fasciitis.	304 (295)	182	–
8. Calcitonin.	307 (297)	72	–
9. Osteoporosis.	308 (298)	77	–
10. Rickety rosary.	311 (301)	74	–
11. Paget's disease of bone (2).	317 (307)	84	–
12. Complications of Paget's disease.	317 (307)	84	–
13. Kienböck's disease.	318 (308)	111	–

14.	Perthes' disease (2).	318 (308)	111	–
15.	Torticollis.	321 (311)	156	–
16.	Cervical rib.	322 (312)	155	–
17.	Diagnosis of slipped capital femoral epiphysis.	323 (313)	175	Aug 13
18.	Genu valgum (3).	324 (314)	177	–
19.	Knock knee.	324 (314)	177	–
20.	Pes planus.	326 (316)	183	–
21.	Hallux valgus.	327 (317)	184	–
22.	Ideal stump.	329 (319)	335	–
23.	Below knee amputation.	329 (319)	334	–
24.	Arthroscopy.	334 (324)	190	–

SHORT ANSWERS

1.	Dupuytren's contracture.	302 (293)	164	–
2.	Tennis elbow.	302 (293)	158	Aug 15
3.	Name the nerves injured in the following situations: a. Medial epicondylitis. b. Tennis elbow.	302 (293)	–, 158	–
4.	de Quervain's tenosynovitis.	303 (294)	162	–
5.	de Quervain's disease.	303 (294)	162	Aug 14
6.	Ganglion (2).	303 (294)	162	Feb 15
7.	Carpal tunnel syndrome.	303 (294)	163	Aug 14
8.	Calcaneal spur.	– (–)	182	–
9.	Exostosis (2).	317 (307)	26, 120	–
10.	Radiological features of Paget's disease.	317 (307)	84	Aug 13
11.	Name the osteochondritis of the following: a. Femoral head. b. Lunate bone.	318 (308)	110, 111	–
12.	Torticollis.	321 (311)	156	Aug 14
13.	Bryant's triangle.	– (–)	176	–

14.	Genu valgum.	324 (314)	177	-
15.	Causes:			
	a. Pes planus.			
	b. Pes cavus.	326, - (316, -)	183, -	-
16.	Guillotine amputation.	328 (318)	333	-
17.	Phantom limb.	330 (320)	336	-
18.	Orthosis.	332 (322)	336	Feb 15
19.	Preservation of amputated finger for transfer to a referral center.	- (-)	-	Feb 13

BIBLIOGRAPHY

1. Maheshwari, Mhaskar. Essential Orthopaedics, 5th edition. New Delhi: Jaypee Brothers Medical Publishers (P) Ltd; 2015.
2. Mayil Vahanan Natarajan. Textbook of Orthopaedics and Traumatology, 7th edition. Haryana: Wolters Kluwer Health; 2011.

Section 4

OBSTETRICS

Part I and II

INSTRUCTIONS TO READERS

- Chapterwise based on Sheila Balakrishnan's TEXTBOOK OF OBSTETRICS, 2nd edition (Code: SHLA) with page numbers of answers
- Page numbers of answers from DC Dutta's TEXTBOOK OF OBSTETRICS, 8th edition (Code: DUTTA) has also been mentioned
- The year in which questions have recently appeared (last nine question papers from Aug 2011 to Aug 2015) have been mentioned under the recent year's heading
- The number of times a question has been repeated, between 1990 and 2015, is mentioned within brackets along with the respective questions.

Part I: Basics of Obstetrics
Chapters 1 to 5

1. Anatomy of the Female Reproductive Organs and Pelvis
2. Bony Pelvis
3. Fetus and Fetopelvic Relations
4. Examination of the Pregnant Woman
5. Development of Placenta and Fetus

Part II: Normal Pregnancy
Chapters 6 to 8

6. Maternal Changes in Pregnancy
7. Diagnosis and Features of Normal Pregnancy
8. Antenatal Care

SHORT NOTES

	SHLA	DUTTA	Recent Years
1. Pelvic inlet.	20	99	Aug 14
2. Diagonal conjugate.	22	100	–
3. Diameters of fetal skull (with diagram).	28	96	–
4. Caput succedaneum (2).	33	98	–
5. Cephalhematoma (6).	33	558	Feb 13
6. Fetal circulation.	69	49	–
7. Pregnancy changes in first trimester.	74	52	–
8. Genital tract changes during pregnancy.	74	52	Aug 12
9. Breastfeeding changes in pregnancy.	75	56	–
10. Carbohydrate metabolism in pregnancy.	76	61	–
11. Hematological changes during pregnancy (4).	77	58	Feb 13
12. Cardiovascular system (CVS) changes during pregnancy (2).	79	60	Feb 12, Aug 13
13. Urinary tract changes during pregnancy.	81	63	–
14. Glycosuria in pregnancy.	82	326	–
15. Diagnosis of pregnancy in the first trimester.	88	73	–
16. Antenatal care (2).	93	106	–

SHORT ANSWERS

	SHLA	DUTTA	Recent Years
1. What are the planes of the inlet, midpelvis and outlet in the true pelvis?	20	99	Feb 15
2. Diameters of pelvic inlet.	20	100	Feb 13, Feb 14
3. Diagonal conjugate.	22	100	–

4. Obstetric conjugate and its importance.	22	100	Aug 13
5. Sagittal suture and its importance.	26	95	–
6. Occipitofrontal diameter.	28	96	Aug 14
7. Molding.	31	97	Feb 12
8. Cephalhematoma (2).	33	558	Aug 14
9. Implantation.	57	25	–
10. Hematological changes during pregnancy.	77	58	–
11. Urinary tract changes during pregnancy.	81	63	–
12. Osiander's sign.	88	74	Aug 14
13. Hegar's sign (4).	89	75	Feb 14
14. Pregnancy—diagnosis tests.	89	75	Aug 14
15. Braxton Hicks contraction.	90	54	–
16. Quickening.	90	78	–
17. Mention differential diagnosis for pregnancy.	91	81	Aug 13
18. Aims of antenatal care (2).	93	106	Aug 15
19. Objectives of antenatal care.	93	106	Feb 14
20. Immunization during pregnancy (2).	94	113	Feb 13
21. Enumerate danger signs in pregnancy.	96	111	–
22. Preconceptional counseling.	97	116	–
23. Importance of prenatal care.	97	116	–

Part III and IV

Part III: Normal Labor
Chapters 9 to 11

9. Mechanism of Normal Labor
10. Onset and Stages of Labor
11. Conduct of Normal Labor

Part IV: Abnormal Pregnancy
Chapters 12 to 24

12. Antepartum Hemorrhage
13. Hyperemesis Gravidarum
14. a. Spontaneous Abortion or Miscarriage
    b. Recurrent Miscarriage or Recurrent Pregnancy Loss
15. Ectopic Pregnancy
16. Gestational Trophoblastic Disease
17. Multiple Pregnancy
18. Preterm Labor and Premature Rupture of Membranes
19. Intrauterine Growth Restriction
20. Late Intrauterine Fetal Death
21. Disorders of Amniotic Fluid Volume
22. Prolonged Pregnancy
23. Gynecological Problems in Pregnancy
24. Abnormalities of the Placenta and Cord

	SHLA	DUTTA	Recent Years
ESSAYS			
1. Define normal labor and stages of labor. Write the mechanism and management of normal labor (2).	100, 115	134, 138	–
2. Define antepartum hemorrhage (APH). Discuss the etiology, types, clinical			

features, differential diagnosis and management of placenta previa at 32 weeks of gestation.	128	282	Feb 12
3. Define APH. What are its causes? How do you diagnose and manage a case of placenta previa (3)?	128	282	-
4. Define APH. Discuss diagnosis and management of abruptio placentae. Mention the complications (6).	128, 133	282, 294	-
5. Discuss etiology and types of placenta previa. How would you manage a third gravida with 32 weeks of pregnancy with posterior placenta previa (5)?	128	282	-
6. A 22-year-old second gravida presents with history of 8 months of amenorrhea and bleeding per vaginam (PV). How will you proceed?	129	282	-
7. Discuss the diagnosis, management and complications of accidental hemorrhage.	133	294	-
8. Primigravida with 36 weeks of gestation with BP 140/100 with painful bleeding PV. Discuss diagnosis, investigations, management and complications.	135	294	Aug 14
9. Primigravida with 20 years, has come to hospital with bleeding PV at 8 months of amenorrhea. What are the differential diagnoses? Discuss the management of abruptio placentae and its complications.	136	297	-
10. Describe the etiology, clinical features and management of a case of hyperemesis gravidarum (4).	141	181	-
11. What are the causes of second trimester abortions? How do you diagnose and manage a case of cervical incompetence (2)?	148	187, 197	-

12.	Discuss the differential diagnosis and management of acute ectopic gestation (3).	161	207	-
13.	Define vesicular mole. Discuss the signs, symptoms and diagnosis of vesicular mole. What are the complications of vesicular mole? How do you follow-up a case of vesicular mole after evacuation (5)?	169	222	-
14.	Define multiple pregnancy. Discuss the etiology, diagnosis, complications and management of twin gestation during pregnancy.	178	233	Aug 12
15.	Discuss types of twins, maternal and fetal complications in multiple pregnancy. Elaborate on the diagnosis and management of a primigravida at 36 weeks, who is diagnosed to have twin pregnancy. Brief on intra- and postpartum management.	178	233	Feb 14
16.	Discuss the diagnosis, complications and management of twin pregnancy (4).	180	236	-
17.	Define preterm labor. Explain the etiology and management of preterm labor (2).	192	365	Feb 13
18.	Define intrauterine growth restriction. Describe the etiology, diagnosis and management of intrauterine growth restriction.	201	533	-
19.	Describe the causes, diagnosis and management of intrauterine fetal death (IUFD) (4).	208	375	-

SHORT NOTES

1.	First stage of labor.	108	140	Feb 12
2.	Normal second stage of labor.	111	143	-
3.	Differentiate true from false labor pain.	113	137	-

4. Partograph (2).	121	607	Feb 14
5. Partogram.	121	607	Aug 15
6. What is partogram? How do you monitor a patient in labor?	121	607	-
7. What is alert line, action line and their importance?	121	607	Aug 13
8. How will one differentiate antepartum hemorrhage due to placenta previa from abruptio placentae?	128, 133	287	Feb 15
9. Couvelaire uterus (4).	135	296	-
10. Signs and symptoms of abruptio placentae.	135	297	Feb 14
11. Coagulation failure in obstetrics (2).	137	711	-
12. Hyperemesis gravidarum (2).	141	181	Aug 12 Feb 13
13. Enumerate the causes of first trimester pregnancy loss.	145	187	Feb 15
14. Inevitable abortion (2).	145	189	-
15. Incomplete abortion (2).	145	190	-
16. Missed abortion (9).	146	190	Aug 12 Aug 14
17. Septic abortion.	146	191	-
18. Recurrent abortion (2).	148	195	Feb 13
19. Habitual abortion	148	195	-
20. Etiology and investigations of recurrent abortion.	148	195	Aug 13
21. Cervical incompetence (4).	149	197	-
22. Cerclage stitch.	150	199	-
23. Differential diagnosis of ruptured ectopic pregnancy (2).	161	212	-
24. Medical management of unruptured ectopic pregnancy.	162	216	-
25. Follow-up of vesicular mole.	171	227	Aug 12 Aug 14
26. Enumerate the complications encountered during pregnancy and labor in multiple pregnancy (3).	180	237	-

27. Complications of multiple pregnancy.	180	237	–
28. Conjoint twins.	185	244, 473	Feb 12
29. Diagnosis of multiple pregnancy.	186	236	–
30. Delivery of second twin—in transverse lie with cord prolapse.	189	242	–
31. Prematurity (2).	–	528	–
32. Preterm labor (2).	192	365	–
33. Diagnosis and management of preterm labor.	193	366	Feb 14
34. Prevention of preterm labor.	194	366	Feb 12
35. Intrauterine growth restriction.	201	533	–
36. Intrauterine death.	208	375	Aug 12
37. Ultrasonographic findings in IUFD.	209	376	–
38. Polyhydramnios (2).	213	246	–
39. Causes of hydramnios and its management.	213	246	Aug 14
40. Oligohydramnios.	215	250	–
41. Prolonged pregnancy—etiology.	218	371	Aug 12
42. Postmaturity.	218	371	–
43. Complications of postmaturity.	218	374	–
44. Fibroid complicating pregnancy.	221	359	–
45. Placenta succenturiata.	226	251	–
46. What is bad obstetric history (BOH)? Enumerate the causes of BOH.	–	399	–

SHORT ANSWERS

1. Define normal labor.	100	134	–
2. Engagement.	102	91, 145	Aug 12
3. Restitution.	105	148	Feb 12
4. Cervical ripening.	107	599	Aug 12
5. False labor pains.	113	137	–
6. Complications of artificial rupture of membrane (ARM) (2).	116	601	Aug 13
7. Active management of third stage of labor (2).	119	164	Feb 14 Feb 15

8.	Prophylactic methergine.	119	164	Aug 13
9.	Couvelaire uterus.	135	296	Feb 12
10.	Complications of abruptio placentae.	136	297	Aug 12
11.	Etiology of hyperemesis.	141	181	–
12.	Inevitable abortion.	145	189	–
13.	Incomplete abortion.	145	190	–
14.	What is incomplete abortion and management?	145	190	Aug 13
15.	Missed abortion.	146	190	–
16.	Diagnosis and management of missed abortion.	146	190	Feb 14
17.	Recurrent abortions.	148	195	Feb 12
18.	Encerclage.	150	199	Feb 12
19.	Decidual cast.	158	209	–
20.	Criteria for medical management of ectopic pregnancy.	162	216	Feb 13
21.	Follow-up postvesicular mole evacuation.	171	227	Feb 13
22.	Enumerate the antenatal complications encountered in multiple pregnancies.	180	237	Feb 15
23.	Define prematurity. Mention two complications.	–	528	–
24.	Define polyhydramnios and oligohydramnios.	213, 215	246, 250	Aug 13
25.	Battledore placenta.	227	253	Aug 14
26.	Causes of BOH.	–	399	–
27.	Causes of lower abdominal pain during pregnancy.	–	355	–

Part V and VI

Part V: Medical Disorders in Pregnancy

Chapters 25 to 36

Part VI: Special Situations

Chapters 37 and 38

	SHLA	DUTTA	Recent Years
ESSAYS			
1. Explain briefly the principles in management of labor in heart disease complicating pregnancy (3).	232	321	-
2. Define gestation diabetes mellitus (GDM). Discuss the indications for screening and methods of screening for GDM. Elaborate on management of Mrs X, G3 P2 L2 diagnosed to have GDM at 32 weeks of pregnancy. Brief on maternal/fetal complications.	240	326	Feb 14

3. Classify hypertensive disorders in pregnancy. Etiopathogenesis and clinical features, complications of preeclampsia and management of eclampsia.	252	255	Feb 13
4. How do you investigate and treat a case of anemia in pregnancy (6)?	284	303	–
5. What are the causes of anemia? How will you manage a term pregnant lady with 6 g% hemoglobin (Hb)?	284	303	–
6. A primi with 26 weeks of pregnancy presents with hemoglobin of 7 g. Discuss investigations and management in pregnancy and in labor.	284	303	Aug 13

SHORT NOTES

1. Management of labor in heart disease complicating pregnancy.	232	321	–
2. Neonatal complications in a diabetic mother.	243	329	Aug 13
3. Gestational diabetes.	244	326	Aug 12
4. Screening test for gestational diabetes (4).	244	326	Feb 13
5. GDM diagnosis and management.	244	326	Aug 15
6. Oral glucose tolerance test using 75 g glucose.	244	327	Feb 15
7. Oral glucose challenge test.	245	326	Aug 14
8. Imminent eclampsia.	259	–	–
9. HELLP syndrome.	259	258	Aug 14
10. Antepartum eclampsia (3).	266	268	Feb 14
11. Magnesium sulfate ($MgSO_4$) therapy in obstetrics.	268	273, 583	Aug 13
12. Asymptomatic bacteriuria.	273	347	–
13. Anemia in pregnancy—prevention.	286, 289	308	–
14. Trichomonas vaginitis (4).	300	356	–
15. Acquired immunodeficiency syndrome (AIDS) infection (3).	302	350	–

16.	Prevention of vertical transmission of human immunodeficiency virus (HIV) in pregnancy.	303	351	Feb 14
17.	Erythroblastosis fetalis.	307	388	–
18.	Rh isoimmunization (2).	307	386	–
19.	Deep vein thrombosis.	317	508	–
20.	Vaginal birth after cesarean (VBAC) section.	339	384	Feb 13
21.	Complications in a grand multipara during pregnancy and labor.	344	398	–

SHORT ANSWERS

1.	Infective endocarditis prophylaxis in labor.	231	322	Feb 14
2.	Oral glucose challenge test.	245	326	–
3.	Define pregnancy-induced hypertension (PIH). Classify hypertensive diseases in pregnancy.	252	255, 256	Feb 15
4.	Definition of eclampsia.	253	268	Aug 12
5.	Pathogenesis of preeclampsia.	254	257	–
6.	HELLP syndrome (2).	259	258	–
7.	Mention complications of eclampsia.	260	271	–
8.	Differential diagnosis of convulsions during pregnancy.	267	270	–
9.	$MgSO_4$ in eclampsia (2).	268	273	Feb 12 Aug 12
10.	Asymptomatic bacteriuria (2).	273	347	Aug 14
11.	Causes for renal failure in obstetrics.	277	707	–
12.	Classification of anemia in pregnancy.	284	303	–
13.	Prophylactic iron therapy.	287	308	Feb 14
14.	Universal precautions to be observed in treating HIV patient (2).	306	–	–
15.	Prevention of Rh isoimmunization (2).	310	389	Feb 14
16.	Prophylaxis of Rh isoimmunization.	310	389	Aug 12

17. Causes for coagulation disorder in obstetrics.	317	711	Aug 14
18. Scar dehiscence (2).	338	496	Feb 12 Aug 12
19. VBAC.	339	384	Feb 12 Aug 12
20. Complications of VBAC.	339	385	–
21. Why should we cut short second stage of labor in severe PIH?	–	–	–

Part VII and VIII

Part VII: Abnormal Labor
Chapters 39 to 47

39. Abnormal or Dysfunctional Labor
40. Abnormal Uterine Action
41. Contracted Pelvis and Cephalopelvic Disproportion
42. Malpositions and Malpresentations
43. Other Fetal Problems Leading to Dystocia
44. Obstructed Labor
45. Third Stage Complications
46. Uterine Rupture
47. Other Injuries to the Parturient Canal

Part VIII: Puerperium
Chapters 48 to 50

48. Normal Puerperium
49. Lactation and Breastfeeding
50. Abnormal Puerperium

	SHLA	DUTTA	Recent Years
ESSAYS			
1. Discuss the causes and management of unengaged head in primi at term.	364	93	-
2. Describe the etiology, diagnosis and management of right occipitoposterior (ROP)? (2)	365	424	-
3. How will you diagnose the ROP clinically? Discuss the mechanism of labor in ROP in: a. Anthropoid pelvis. b. Android pelvis and its management in each condition.	365	424	-

4. What is deep transverse arrest? Mention how you diagnose and treat such case (6).	369	431	-
5. A primigravida woman has come at 37 weeks of gestation with no risk factors other than breech presentation. Describe how one should plan for her mode of delivery. What procedure could be done to facilitate normal delivery?	375	434	Feb 15
6. What are the causes of breech presentation? How do you manage breech presentation at 34–36 weeks of pregnancy?	375	435	-
7. Describe the causes, diagnosis and management of breech presentation (5).	375	435	-
8. Discuss etiology, diagnosis and management of a case of transverse lie at term in early labor.	383	454	-
9. What is obstructed labor? Write causes and treatment (3).	393	467	-
10. What are the causes for third stage complications? Explain the management of atonic postpartum hemorrhage.	395	474	-
11. Define postpartum hemorrhage. What are the types of postpartum hemorrhage? Discuss in detail the predisposing factors, clinical features and management of atonic postpartum hemorrhage.	395	474	Aug 12
12. Define postpartum hemorrhage. Discuss the management and complications.	395	474	Aug 14
13. Describe the etiology, diagnosis and management of postpartum hemorrhage (3).	395	474	-

14. What are the causes of ruptured uterus? Discuss signs and symptoms of obstructed labor and their management.	410, 393	494, 467	Aug 13
15. What are the causes of ruptured uterus? How will you diagnose and treat such case (4).	410	494	–
16. What is puerperium? Describe the complications of puerperium and its management.	422, 433	168, 500	Feb 12
17. Discuss the etiology, clinical features and management of puerperal infection (6).	433	500	–

SHORT NOTES

1. Hypotonic uterine inertia.	357	416	–
2. Incoordinate uterine action (2).	357	417	–
3. Difference between retraction ring and contraction ring dystocia.	358	421	–
4. Assessment of cephalopelvic disproportion.	362	410	–
5. Trial labor (3).	363	412	–
6. Face to pubis delivery (2).	368	428	–
7. Deep transverse arrest (4).	369	431	Aug 12 Feb 13 Aug 14 Aug 15
8. Management of aftercoming head of breech presentation (3).	380	444	–
9. Delivery of aftercoming head.	380	444	Aug 14
10. Shoulder presentation.	383	454	–
11. Cord prolapse (2).	385	460	–
12. Shoulder dystocia (2).	390	469	Feb 14
13. Hydrocephalus (2).	392	470	–
14. Bandl's ring.	393	420	–
15. Management and complications of third stage of labor (2).	119, 395	162, 474	–

16.	Third stage complication.	395	474	–
17.	Atonic postpartum hemorrhage (PPH) (6).	395	474	–
18.	Define atonic PPH and its management.	395	474	Aug 15
19.	Vulval hematoma.	396	492	Feb 12
20.	Internal iliac ligation.	400	483	Feb 12
21.	Retained placenta.	403	484	–
22.	Adherent placenta.	404	484	–
23.	Placenta accreta.	404	486	–
24.	Inversion of uterus.	406	487	–
25.	Acute inversion of uterus (2).	406	487	Feb 14
26.	Prevention of uterine rupture.	412	498	–
27.	Complete perineal tear (3).	414	489	Feb 13
28.	Management of complete perineal tear.	414	490	Aug 14
29.	Physiology of lactation.	427	173	–
30.	Mention the two hormones involved in milk secretion and milk ejection. Enumerate the advantages of breastfeeding.	427, 430	173, 520	–
31.	Breastfeeding (2).	428	519	–
32.	Baby-friendly hospital.	428	519	–
33.	Puerperal pyrexia.	433	500	–
34.	Predisposing causes of puerperal sepsis.	433	501	–
35.	Puerperal sepsis.	433	500	Feb 13

SHORT ANSWERS

1.	Secondary arrest of labor.	351	464	–
2.	Uterine inertia.	357	416	Feb 12
3.	Muller-Munro-Kerr method.	362	411	Feb 12
4.	Causes of mobile head at term (2).	364	93	Feb 13
5.	Causes of unengaged head at term.	364	93	–
6.	Causes of breech presentation.	375	435	–

7.	Causes of difficulty in delivery of aftercoming head in breech.	380	448	–
8.	Delivery of aftercoming head.	380	444	Feb 12
9.	Causes of obstructed labor (2).	393	467	Feb 14
10.	Bandl's ring (4).	393	420	Aug 12 Aug 14
11.	Define postpartum hemorrhage.	395	474	Aug 13
12.	Placenta percreta.	404	–	Feb 12
13.	Define puerperium.	422	168	Aug 12
14.	Complications in puerperium.	433	500	Aug 14
15.	Causes of puerperal pyrexia.	433	500	–
16.	Puerperal pyrexia.	433	500	–
17.	Precipitate labor (3).	–	420	Aug 12

Part IX to XIV

Part IX: Operative Obstetrics

Chapters 51 to 54

Part X: Special Investigations

Chapters 55 to 58

Part XI: Neonatology

Chapters 59 to 61

Part XII: Miscellaneous Topics

Chapters 62 to 64

Part XIII: Contemporary Issues

Chapters 65

Part XIV: Maternal Mortality
Chapters 66

66. Maternal Mortality

	SHLA	DUTTA	Recent Years
ESSAYS			
1. Define cesarean section and its various indications. Explain the management of previous lower segment cesarean section in labor.	458, 339	669, 383	–
2. Enumerate the indications for lower segment cesarean section. Discuss the management of a case of previous cesarean section posted for vaginal delivery.	458, 339	669, 383	–
3. What is induction of labor? What are the indications and methods used for inducing labor (3)?	558	598	–
4. What is induction of labor? Discuss briefly the indications, contraindications and methods of induction of labor.	558	598	Aug 15
SHORT NOTES			
1. Forceps in obstetrics.	443	651	–
2. Complications of forceps application.	444	659	Aug 14
3. Indications for forceps in modern obstetrics.	444	654	–
4. Outlet forceps (5).	444	653	–
5. Suction cup delivery.	447	660	Feb 14
6. Advantages of ventouse over forceps.	449	661	Feb 12
7. External cephalic version (3).	451	663	Aug 13
8. Episiotomy.	453	647	Aug 13
9. Describe the procedure of 'manual removal of the placenta.'	455	478	Feb 15

10.	Craniotomy.	456	666	–
11.	Indications for elective cesarean section.	458	670	–
12.	Enumerate the steps in lower segment cesarean section. Mention some complications of cesarean section (2).	460, 464	671, 677	–
13.	Classical cesarean section.	462	676	–
14.	Complications of emergency cesarean section.	464	677	–
15.	Ultrasonography (USG) in obstetrics (4).	474	732	Feb 12
16.	Ultrasound in first trimester (3).	475	734	Aug 12
17.	If last menstrual period (LMP) is not known, describe the methods by which expected date of delivery (EDD) could be arrived at.	475	734	Feb 15
18.	Anencephaly.	487	471, 736	–
19.	Hydrops fetalis.	493	388	–
20.	Techniques of prenatal diagnosis.	502	129	Feb 12
21.	Reactive non-stress test (NST).	509	122	Aug 13
22.	Biophysical profile.	510	121	Aug 12
23.	Diagnosis of fetal distress.	517	692	–
24.	Monitoring uterine activity during labor.	518	692	Feb 12
25.	Fetal distress in labor.	525	692	–
26.	Care of newborn.	532	517	–
27.	Birth asphyxia.	534	541	Feb 13
28.	Asphyxia neonatorum (2).	534	541	–
29.	Neonatal resuscitation.	534	546	–
30.	APGAR*.	535	543	–
31.	Physiological jaundice.	543	551	–
32.	Neonatal jaundice (4).	543	551	–
33.	Causes of neonatal hyperbilirubinemia.	543	552	Feb 14

*APGAR, 'activity, pulse, grimace, appearance, respiration.'

34.	Respiratory distress syndrome.	549	547	–
35.	Neonatal convulsions (2).	550	557	–
36.	Meconium aspiration syndrome (MAS).	550	550	Aug 15
37.	Birth injuries to child.	552	558	–
38.	Perinatal mortality (4).	554	687	–
39.	Causes of early neonatal deaths and prevention.	555	690	–
40.	Mention indications, contraindications and complications of induction of labor.	558, 562	598	–
41.	Bishop score.	559	600	–
42.	Drugs used for cervical ripening.	560	599	Feb 13
43.	Oxytocin.	566	573	–
44.	Syntocinon in obstetrics.	566	573	–
45.	Prostaglandins.	567	578	–
46.	Antihypertensive drugs in pregnancy.	573	581	–
47.	Epidural anesthesia.	583	593	–
48.	Safe motherhood initiative.	594	680	–
49.	Maternal mortality (5).	594	683	Aug 12
50.	Definition and causes of maternal mortality.	594, 596	683, 685	Feb 14
51.	Causes of maternal mortality.	596	685	Aug 13
52.	Reproductive and child health (RCH) interventions.	–	682	–
53.	Criteria of maternal mortality.	–	–	Aug 13

SHORT ANSWERS

1.	Outlet forceps.	444	653	Aug 12
2.	Indications for outlet forceps.	444	654	Feb 13
3.	Prerequisites for application of outlet forceps.	444	654	–
4.	What are the complications of suction evacuation?	447	663	Aug 13
5.	Chignon	–	–	–
6.	Advantages of vacuum.	449	661	–

7.	External cephalic version (ECV).	451	663	–
8.	Definition and indication for ECV.	451	663	Feb 14
9.	Indication for internal podalic version.	452	665	–
10.	Manual removal of placenta.	455	478	Aug 12
11.	Advantages of elective cesarean section (2).	462	676	–
12.	Write four advantages of LSCS* over classical section.	462	676	–
13.	Indications for classical cesarean section (2).	463	676	Aug 13
14.	Indications for cesarean hysterectomy.	463	678	Feb 13
15.	Any four indications for ultrasound in obstetrics.	475	734	Feb 13
16.	Anencephaly.	487	471, 736	Aug 14
17.	NST (2).	509	122	Aug 15
18.	Causes of birth asphyxia (2).	534	542	Aug 15
19.	APGAR score.	535	543	Aug 15
20.	MAS.	550	550	–
21.	Prevention of perinatal mortality.	555	688	–
22.	Indication of induction of labor (2).	558	598	–
23.	Mifepristone (2).	561	629, 601, 203	Feb 12
24.	Write the dose of oxytocin in induction of labor and in postpartum hemorrhage.	561, 398	575, 477	Aug 13
25.	Complications of induction of labor.	562	598	–
26.	Prostaglandins.	567	578	Aug 15
27.	Contraindications for prostaglandins.	568	579	–
28.	Antihypertensives used in pregnancy.	573	581	–
29.	Pudendal block (2).	581	594	Feb 12 Aug 12
30.	Define maternal mortality and perinatal mortality rates.	594, 554	683, 687	Feb 15

*LSCS, lower segment cesarean section.

31.	Causes of maternal mortality.	596	685	–
32.	RCH interventions.	–	682	Feb 12
33.	Indication for cervicotomy.	–	–	–

BIBLIOGRAPHY

1. Sheila Balakrishnan. Textbook of Obstetrics, 2nd edition. Hyderabad: Paras Medical Publishers; 2013.
2. Hiralal Konar. DC Dutta's Textbook of Obstetrics, 8th edition. New Delhi: Jaypee Brothers Medical Publishers (P) Ltd; 2015.

Section 5

GYNECOLOGY

Gynecology

INSTRUCTIONS TO READERS

- Chapterwise based on Howkins and Bourne Shaw's TEXTBOOK OF GYNAECOLOGY, 16th edition (Code: SHW) with page numbers of answers from 15th edition have also been mentioned within brackets next to it
- Page numbers of answers from the DC Dutta's TEXTBOOK OF GYNAECOLOGY by Hiralal Konar, 6th edition (Code: DUTTA) has also been mentioned
- Page numbers of answers for certain questions which are found exclusively in DC Dutta's TEXTBOOK OF OBSTETRICS are mentioned within brackets next to it
- The year in which questions have recently appeared (last nine question papers from Aug 2011 to Aug 2015) have been mentioned under the recent year's heading
- The number of times a question has been repeated, between 1990 and 2015, is mentioned within brackets along with the respective questions.

Chapters 1 to 5

1. Anatomy
2. Normal Histology
3. Physiology
4. Puberty, Pediatric and Adolescent Gynecology
5. Perimenopause, Menopause, Premature Menopause and Postmenopausal Bleeding

ESSAYS

	SHW	DUTTA	Recent Years
1. Describe the supports of uterus. Discuss the etiology, differential diagnosis and management of uterovaginal prolapse in a 45-year-old multipara.	18, 349 (18, 331)	201, 303	Aug 14
2. Describe the lymphatic drainage of cervix and etiology, clinical features and management of carcinoma cervix (8).	21, 495 (21, 407)	30, 339	–
3. Define normal menstrual cycle. Discuss phases of normal menstrual cycle.	29 (32)	84	–
4. Explain menstrual cycle. Discuss management of metropathia hemorrhagica in a 40-year-old lady.	29, 341 (32, 302)	84, 188	–
5. What are the causes of postmenopausal bleeding? How do you investigate the case? Mention the treatment of one cause (7).	76 (71)	559	–
6. Define postmenopausal bleeding. Discuss in detail the etiology, clinical features and management of postmenopausal bleeding.	76 (71)	559	Aug 12

SHORT NOTES

	SHW	DUTTA	Recent Years
1. Anatomy of fallopian tube.	10 (11)	10	–
2. Levator ani.	15 (15)	17	–
3. Pubic diaphragm.	15 (15)	17	–
4. Supports of uterus (8).	18 (18)	201	Aug 13, Aug 15
5. Lymphatic drainage of the cervix.	20 (21)	30	–

6. Pelvic lymphatic drainage.	20 (21)	28	–
7. Graafian follicle.	26 (28)	85	–
8. Ovulation.	28 (30)	92	–
9. Signs of ovulation.	28 (31)	235	–
10. Luteal phase.	30 (33)	91	–
11. Secretory phase of endometrium.	30 (33)	91	–
12. Functional and therapeutic uses of estrogens.	41, 71 (43, 67)	71, 531	–
13. Feedback mechanism.	44 (40)	77	–
14. Menopause (symptoms, management).	67 (63)	59	Aug 13
15. Hormone replacement therapy.	70 (66)	61	Aug 15
16. Tibolone.	73 (69)	63	Aug 14
17. Etiology and investigations of postmenopausal bleeding.	76 (71)	559	Aug 14
18. Postmenopausal bleeding and management.	76 (71)	559	Feb 15
19. Dilatation and curettage (D and C).	76 (72)	585	–

SHORT ANSWERS

1. Clinical significance of pouch of Douglas.	5 (5)	20	–
2. Course of pelvic ureter.	13 (13)	15	Aug 13
3. Perineal body.	16 (17)	20	Feb 14, Feb 12
4. Mention ligament supports of uterus.	18 (18)	202	–
5. Uterine artery (2).	19 (19)	26	Feb 14
6. Lymphatic drainage of vulva.	20 (21)	30	–
7. Lymphatic drainage of cervix.	20 (21)	30	Aug 12
8. Corpus luteum.	28 (31)	87	–
9. Human chorionic gonadotropin (hCG).	40 (42)	527	–
10. Precocious puberty.	59 (56)	51	Feb 12, Feb 14

11.	Hormonal replacement therapy.	70 (66)	61	-
12.	Estrogen replacement therapy—advantages, indications and contraindications (2).	70 (66)	61	-
13.	Estrogen replacement therapy—indications and contraindications.	70 (66)	61	Feb 15
14.	Premature menopause.	74 (70)	64	Feb 13
15.	Causes of postmenopausal bleeding.	76 (71)	559	Aug 13
16.	Differential diagnosis for postmenopausal bleeding.	76 (71)	559	-

Chapters 6 to 10

6. Gynecological Diagnosis
7. Endoscopy in Gynecology
8. Imaging Modalities in Gynecology
9. Malformations of the Female Generative Organs
10. Sexual Development and Development Disorders

SHORT NOTES

	SHW	DUTTA	Recent Years
1. Contribution of Sims to gynecology.	85, 243 (79, 247)	103, 628, 423	-
2. Pap smear (8).	87 (83)	110	Aug 14
3. Laparoscopy in gynecology (2).	93 (485)	121	Feb 13
4. Hysteroscopy (3).	101 (493)	122	Aug 12
5. Indications for hysteroscopy.	102 (494)	122	-
6. Colposcopy.	105 (497)	115	-
7. Hysterosalpingography (HSG) (5).	111 (501)	238, 588	Feb 12, Aug 12, Feb 13
8. Imperforate hymen (2).	129 (96)	41	-
9. Hematocolpos.	130 (96)	41, 450	Aug 14
10. Turner's syndrome (7).	145 (110)	441, 446	Aug 12
11. Hyperprolactinemia.	151, 257, 259 (117, 204, 216)	464, 471	-

SHORT ANSWERS

	SHW	DUTTA	Recent Years
1. Contribution of Sims to gynecology.	83, 84, 243 (79, 204)	103, 628, 423	Aug 15
2. Indication for endometrial biopsy.	90 (85)	120	-
3. Diagnostic laparoscopy.	94 (486)	121	Aug 15

4.	Complications of operative and diagnostic laparoscopy.	100 (492)	619	Feb 12, Aug 12, Feb 14
5.	Indication for hysteroscopy.	102 (494)	621	Feb 15
6.	List four indications for operative hysteroscopy.	103 (495)	621	Feb 14
7.	Colposcopy.	105 (497)	115	Feb 12
8.	Visual inspection of acetowhite areas (VIAs) and visual inspection with Lugol's iodine (VILI)—comment on it.	105 (497)	324	Aug 15
9.	Imperforate hymen.	129 (96)	41	Feb 12, Aug 12
10.	McIndoe operation.	131 (96)	44	-
11.	Turner's syndrome.	145 (110)	441, 446	Feb 12, Aug 14
12.	Testicular feminizing syndrome.	146 (111)	443	Feb 13

Chapters 11 to 14

11. Sexually Transmitted Diseases
12. Inflammation of the Cervix and Uterus
13. Pelvic Inflammatory Disease
14. Tuberculosis of the Genital Tract

ESSAYS

	SHW	DUTTA	Recent Years
1. Discuss etiopathogenesis of pelvic inflammatory diseases (PIDs). How do you manage chronic pelvic tuberculosis (2)?	177, 191 (445, 158)	127, 140	–
2. Describe the etiology, clinical features and management of acute salpingitis.	177 (445)	170	–
3. Describe the etiology and diagnosis of a case of genital tuberculosis. Mention the management (2).	187 (154)	137	–
4. Describe the pathology, diagnosis and treatment of genital tuberculosis.	187 (154)	137	Aug 11
5. How do you diagnose endometrial tuberculosis? Discuss the treatment of endometrial tuberculosis in a 28-year-old patient.	187 (154)	137	–

SHORT NOTES

	SHW	DUTTA	Recent Years
1. Pelvic abscess.	162 (144)	175	–
2. Trichomonas vaginitis.	163 (145)	163	Aug 13
3. Trichomoniasis.	163 (145)	163	–
4. Candidal vaginitis (2).	164, 383 (146)	164	–
5. Monilial vaginitis.	164, 383 (146)	164	–
6. Erosion cervix (2).	171 (324)	267	–

7.	Treatment of chronic cervicitis.	172 (324)	168	–
8.	Definition and management of PID.	177, 183 (445, 452)	127, 132	–
9.	Chronic PID causes and management.	177 (445, 452)	136	–
10.	Etiology of PID.	177 (445)	128	–
11.	Hydrosalpinx (2).	180 (448)	170	–
12.	Differential diagnosis of PID.	182 (451)	131	–
13.	Asherman's syndrome (2).	190, 250 (210, 156)	459	Aug 14

SHORT ANSWERS

1.	Management of genital herpes.	158 (140)	152	Aug 14
2.	Pelvic abscess.	162 (144)	175	–
3.	Trichomonas vaginalis.	163 (145)	163	Aug 15
4.	Trichomonas vaginitis.	163 (145)	163	–
5.	Candidiasis.	164, 383 (146)	164	Aug 12
6.	Laboratory tests for human immunodeficiency virus (HIV).	166 (148)	155	–
7.	Cervical erosion (2).	171 (324)	267	Aug 12
8.	Chronic cervicitis (2).	171 (324)	167	Feb 12
9.	Pyometra (2).	176 (324)	168	Feb 13
10.	Causes of pyometra.	176 (324)	169	–
11.	Organisms, which cause PID.	177 (445)	129	–
12.	Differential diagnosis for acute salpingitis.	182 (450)	131	–
13.	Differential diagnosis of chronic PID.	183 (451)	–	Aug 14
14.	Tuberculous salpingitis.	188 (154)	137	Feb 12
15.	HSG findings in genital tuberculosis.	191 (157)	141	–
16.	CA-125.	192, 450 (159)	377	–

Chapters 15 to 20

15. Injuries of the Female Genital Tract
16. Injuries to the Intestinal Tract
17. Diseases of the Urinary System
18. Genital Fistulae and Urinary Incontinence
19. Infertility and Sterility
20. Birth Control and Medical Termination of Pregnancy

ESSAYS

	SHW	DUTTA	Recent Years
1. What are the main causes of infertility? How will you investigate a couple with primary infertility? Discuss the management of anovulation as the cause of infertility.	242, 249, 257 (202, 203, 216)	227, 231, 243	Feb 12
2. How will you evaluate the couple with infertility?	242, 250 (203, 211)	231	–
3. Enumerate the causes of secondary infertility. How do you manage the case of secondary infertility (2)?	242, 249 (202)	227, 241	–
4. Enumerate the causes of male and female infertility. Discuss the tests for ovulation. Discuss the seminal analysis.	242, 249, 255, 243 (202, 15, 203)	227, 235, 232	–
5. How will you diagnose ovulatory causes for infertility? Discuss the management of anovulatory infertility.	255 (210, 216)	235, 243	–

6.	How do you investigate a case of female sterility? Enumerate causes (4).	249 (211, 209)	234, 229	–
7.	A young, newly married couple wants contraceptive advice. Describe briefly the various methods, which can be advised to them evaluating the advantages and disadvantages.	263 (222)	500	–
8.	Mention the various methods of contraception. Discuss the advantages and disadvantages of oral contraceptives.	263, 273 (222, 231)	475, 485	–
9.	Discuss the mechanism of action and complications of IUCD* (2).	270 (229)	479	–
10.	What are the different types of hormonal contraceptives? Discuss the advantages and disadvantages of injectable contraceptives.	273, 276 (231, 234)	485, 491	–

SHORT NOTES

1.	Stress incontinence (2).	224 (188)	398	–
2.	Male infertility (2).	240 (201)	228	–
3.	Secondary infertility causes and investigations.	240 (201)	227	Aug 15
4.	How do you investigate male infertility?	242 (201)	231	–
5.	Semen analysis (6).	243 (203)	232	–
6.	Huhner postcoital test.	243 (204)	239, 115	–
7.	Postcoital test (2).	243 (204)	239, 115	Feb 13
8.	Evaluation of tubal factor infertility (2).	251 (211)	237	–
9.	Tubal patency test (5).	251 (211)	237	Feb 14
10.	Hysteroscopy in infertility.	253 (213)	238	Feb 12

*IUCD, intrauterine contraceptive device.

11.	Tests for ovulation (4).	255 (215)	235	Aug 12
12.	Basal body temperature.	255 (215)	235	–
13.	Induction of ovulation (2).	257 (217)	243	Aug 15
14.	Barrier contraceptives.	266 (224)	476	–
15.	IUCD (10).	269 (227)	479	Aug 13
16.	Multiload Copper T.	269 (227)	480	–
17.	Copper T 380A.	269 (227)	480	–
18.	Missed IUCD.	271 (229)	484	Feb 12
19.	Complications of IUCDs (2).	271 (229)	482	–
20.	Complications of Copper T insertion.	271 (229)	482	–
21.	Mirena.	272 (230)	480	Feb 14
22.	Hormonal contraception (2).	273 (231)	485	–
23.	Oral contraception (3).	273 (231)	485	–
24.	Non-contraceptive benefits of hormonal contraceptives.	273 (231)	489	–
25.	Contraindications for combined oral pill.	275 (231)	487	–
26.	Low-dose pills for contraception.	275 (233)	491	–
27.	Injectable contraception.	276 (234)	491	Feb 12
28.	Subdermal implant—Norplant.	277 (234)	492	–
29.	Postcoital contraception.	279 (236)	492	–
30.	Emergency contraception (3).	279 (236)	492	Aug 12
31.	Surgical method of contraception.	280 (238)	494	–
32.	Vasectomy (2).	280 (238)	494	Aug 14
33.	Puerperal sterilization.	281 (239)	495	–
34.	Interval sterilization.	282 (239)	495	–
35.	Minilap technique (6).	282 (240)	497	Feb 14, Feb 15
36.	Laparoscopic sterilization (2).	283 (241)	498	Aug 11
37.	Complications of tubal ligation.	284 (242)	499	–
38.	Medical Termination of Pregnancy (MTP) Act (2).	286 (244)	– (202)	–
39.	MTP in first trimester (4).	288 (245)	– (203)	Aug 15

40.	What are the methods for first trimester MTP? Write about menstrual regulation.	288 (245)	– (203, 646)	–
41.	Menstrual regulation (3).	288 (245)	– (646)	–
42.	Methods available for MTP in less than 6 weeks of pregnancy.	288 (245)	– (203)	–
43.	Complications of first trimester MTP.	289 (247)	– (206)	–
44.	Complications of MTP.	289, 291 (247, 248)	– (206)	–
45.	Mention the methods of MTP in the second trimester of pregnancy.	290 (247)	– (204)	–

SHORT ANSWERS

1.	Rectovaginal fistula.	207 (172)	427	Feb 13
2.	Causes for retention of urine.	211 (175)	409	–
3.	Causes of acute retention of urine (2).	211 (175)	409	Feb 14
4.	Causes for retention of urine in: a. Reproductive women. b. Pubertal age.	211 (175)	409	–
5.	Diagnosis of genitourinary fistula.	221 (185)	419	–
6.	Methylene blue—three swab test.	221 (186)	419	Aug 14
7.	Causes of dyspareunia (2).	239 (199)	568	–
8.	Postcoital test (2).	243 (204)	115	Feb 15
9.	Rubin's cannula.	251 (211)	238	Feb 12
10.	Sonosalpingography.	253 (213)	239	–
11.	Basal body temperature.	255 (215)	235	Feb 13, Aug 14
12.	Management of luteal phase defect.	257, 259 (57, 218)	237, 247, 253, 536	Aug 13
13.	Femshield.	267 (226)	476	–
14.	Today.	268 (226)	478	–
15.	Contraindications for IUCD (3).	270 (228)	480	Aug 14

16.	Advantages of IUCD.	272 (230)	484	Aug 12
17.	Benefits of combined pills contraceptives.	273 (231)	488	–
18.	Non-contraceptive beneficial effects of oral contraceptive pill.	273 (231)	489	Aug 13
19.	Triphasic pills.	275 (233)	490	–
20.	Mini pill.	275 (233)	491	Feb 13
21.	Norplant.	277 (235)	492	Aug 14
22.	Emergency contraception (2).	279 (236)	492	Feb 14
23.	Postcoital contraception.	279 (236)	492	–
24.	What are estrogen-free pills?	279 (237)	493	–
25.	Mifepristone.	279 (237)	537, 493	Aug 12
26.	Laparoscopic sterilization.	283 (241)	498	–
27.	Menstrual regulation.	288 (245)	– (646)	Aug 12
28.	First trimester MTP.	288 (245)	– (203)	Feb 13, Aug 13
29.	Second trimester MTP.	290 (247)	– (204)	Feb 12

Chapters 21 to 26

21. Ectopic Gestation
22. Gestational Trophoblastic Diseases
23. Disorders of Menstruation—Amenorrhea
24. Menorrhagia
25. Genital Prolapse
26. Displacements

ESSAYS

	SHW	DUTTA	Recent Years
1. Discuss the etiology, clinical features and management of tubal pregnancy (3).	294, 299, 304 (266, 271, 276)	- (208)	-
2. Discuss the differential diagnosis and management of acute ectopic gestation (3).	301, 304 (273, 276)	- (212)	-
3. Discuss the differential diagnosis of menorrhagia in a 35-year-old woman. Describe hormonal treatment in dysfunctional uterine bleeding (4).	335, 343 (299, 302)	185, 191	-
4. Define dysfunctional uterine bleeding (DUB). Discuss the classification, clinical evaluation, diagnosis, differential diagnosis and treatment of DUB.	- (301)	187	Feb 14
5. Define DUB. What are the different types of DUB? Discuss the management of each one of them (3).	- (301)	187	-
6. Classify genital prolapse. Discuss etiology, clinical features, differential diagnosis and management of nulliparous prolapse.	349 (331)	204	Feb 12, Aug 12

7. Describe pelvic floor. Discuss etiology of prolapse. How will you manage a lady of 55 years with third degree uterovaginal prolapse? Mention the steps of surgery (2).	15, 349, 359 (14, 331, 340)	17, 203, 210	-
8. What are the causes of mass descending per vaginam in a 30-year-old nulliparous woman? How do you manage third-degree uterovaginal prolapse in such patient?	349, 359 (332, 337)	203, 210	-
9. What are the degrees of genital prolapse? Treatment of procidentia in a 80-year-old lady.	350, 356 (332, 341)	205, 210	-

SHORT NOTES

1. Decidual cast.	299 (272)	- (209)	-
2. Medical treatment of ectopic gestation.	304 (276)	- (215)	Feb 13
3. Methotrexate.	304 (276)	513, 516	Aug 13
4. Management of unruptured ectopic pregnancy.	307 (278)	- (216)	Aug 14
5. Cervical pregnancy.	308 (279)	- (220)	Aug 12
6. Ovarian pregnancy.	308 (269)	- (220)	Feb 13
7. Classification of gestational trophoblastic disease (2).	311 (251)	361	-
8. Follow-up of molar pregnancy (postevacuation).	316 (256)	367 (227)	Feb 14
9. Cryptomenorrhea (12).	323 (284)	450	Aug 13, Feb 15
10. Anorexia nervosa.	323 (285)	464	-
11. What is breakthrough bleeding? How do you manage it?	333 (294)	489	-

12.	Metrorrhagia.	333 (294)	186	–
13.	Puberty menorrhagia (2).	339 (301)	54	Aug 12
14.	Metropathia hemorrhagica (5).	341 (302)	188	Feb 13
15.	Cystic glandular hyperplasia (2).	342 (303)	188	–
16.	Nulliparous prolapse (3).	350 (332)	204	–
17.	Procidentia.	351 (332)	206	–
18.	Enterocele.	351, 361 (332, 342)	205	Aug 13
19.	Decubitus ulcer.	354 (335)	206	Feb 14
20.	Urinary symptoms associated with genital prolapse.	355 (336)	208	–
21.	Differential diagnosis of mass per vagina.	355 (336)	210	–
22.	Pessary treatment of prolapse.	356 (337)	210	–
23.	Fothergill's operation.	358 (339)	216	Feb 13
24.	Complications of hysterectomy.	360 (340)	596, 222	–

SHORT ANSWERS

1.	Pelvic hematocele.	300 (272)	–	Feb 12, Aug 12
2.	Culdocentesis.	302, 183 (274, 451)	120	Feb 12
3.	Medical management of unruptured ectopic pregnancy.	307 (278)	- (216)	–
4.	Indications for expectant management of unruptured ectopic pregnancy.	308 (278)	- (216)	–
5.	Follow-up of molar pregnancy (postevacuation) (2).	316 (256)	367 (227)	–
6.	Causes of primary amenorrhea.	322 (284)	451	–
7.	What is cryptomenorrhea?	323 (284)	450	–
8.	Menorrhagia.	335 (299)	185	–
9.	Metropathia hemorrhagica.	341 (302)	188	–
10.	Classification of uterovaginal prolapse.	350 (332)	205	–
11.	Decubitus ulcer (2).	354 (335)	206	Aug 12

12.	Differential diagnosis of mass descending per vagina.	355 (336)	210	Feb 14
13.	Le Fort's repair (2).	360 (341)	221	Aug 12
14.	Complications of vaginal hysterectomy (2).	360 (340)	222	Aug 13
15.	Management of postpill amenorrhea.	– (–)	466	–

Chapters 27 to 32

ESSAYS

	SHW	DUTTA	Recent Years
1. Mention the specific causes of leukorrhea. How do you confirm the diagnosis? Briefly mention the treatment of any one of them.	382 (130)	551	–
2. Mention the types of fibroids. Discuss the various signs and symptoms of a fibroid uterus. How will you manage a 30-year-old infertile lady with fibroid uterus (4)?	392 (352)	273, 276 279	–
3. What are the types of fibroids? Write the clinical features, diagnosis and management of fibroid uterus in 25-year-old woman with infertility.	392 (352)	273, 276	Feb 15
4. Discuss differential diagnosis and investigations of a midline mass of 20 weeks size in a 40-year-old woman. How do you manage a case of fibroid uterus of 20 weeks size in a multiparous woman?	398 (358)	278	–
5. What are the causes of mass per abdomen in a 45-year-old woman? Discuss the types of fibroid. Signs and symptoms, diagnosis and			

	management of fibroid uterus.	398, 392 (358, 352)	278, 273	Aug 13
6.	Define endometriosis. Write diagnosis and management of a case of endometriosis in a 35-year-old lady with one child (3).	409 (465)	304, 308	-
7.	Define endometriosis. Discuss the etiology, pathology, clinical features and management of endometriosis (6).	409 (465)	304	Feb 13
8.	Describe the clinical features, diagnosis and management of pelvic endometriosis.	413 (468)	306	Aug 15

SHORT NOTES

1.	Bartholin's abscess (3).	372 (120)	162	Aug 13
2.	Bartholin's cyst.	377 (125)	162	-
3.	Leukorrhea—investigations and management.	382 (130)	551	Aug 14
4.	Bacterial vaginosis (3).	384 (131)	152	Feb 14
5.	Senile vaginitis.	386 (134)	165	Feb 12
6.	Fibroid polyp.	391 (351)	286	-
7.	Broad ligament fibroid.	392 (352)	273	Feb 14
8.	Submucosal fibroid (2).	392 (352)	273	-
9.	Degeneration of fibroid uterus.	394 (353)	275	-
10.	Red degeneration (8).	395 (355)	275	-
11.	Complications of fibroid uterus (4).	395 (356)	278	-
12.	Hematometra.	398 (357)	41, 450	-
13.	Differential diagnosis of fibroid polyp.	398 (357)	286	-
14.	Myomectomy (3).	401 (360)	281, 604	Aug 12
15.	Chocolate cyst (7).	411 (467)	306	-
16.	Adenomyosis (6).	420 (474)	314	Feb 12, Aug 14
17.	Functional cysts of ovary.	429 (368)	289	-

18.	Polycystic ovarian disease (PCOD) (3).	431 (369)	459, 569	Feb 12, Feb 13, Feb 14

SHORT ANSWERS

1.	Bartholinitis (2).	372 (120)	161	-
2.	Bartholin's abscess.	372 (120)	162	Aug 14
3.	List main causes of pruritus vulva.	373 (121)	553	Aug 13
4.	Bartholin's cyst.	377 (125)	162	Feb 12, Aug 12
5.	Bacterial vaginosis.	384 (131)	152	Feb 13
6.	Clue cells (2).	384 (131)	152	Feb 15
7.	Toxic shock syndrome (2).	388 (135)	166	Aug 14
8.	Unusual forms of leiomyomatosis.	392 (352)	273	-
9.	Red degeneration.	395 (355)	275	Feb 12
10.	Sarcomatous degeneration.	395 (355)	276	Aug 12
11.	Differential diagnosis of fibroid uterus.	398 (357)	278	Aug 14
12.	Prerequisites for myomectomy (2).	401 (360)	282	Feb 14
13.	Etiology of endometriosis.	409 (465)	305	-
14.	Chocolate cysts of ovaries.	411 (467)	306	Feb 14
15.	Medical management of endometriosis (2).	417 (471)	310	-
16.	Clinical features of adenomyosis.	420 (475)	314	Aug 13
17.	Theca lutein cysts of ovary.	430 (369)	290	Aug 13
18.	Diagnosis of PCOD.	431 (369)	459	-

Chapters 33 to 36

33. Ovarian Tumors
34. Breast
35. Acute and Chronic Pelvic Pain
36. Dysmenorrhea, Premenstrual Syndrome

	SHW	DUTTA	Recent Years
ESSAYS			
1. Classify ovarian tumors. Discuss in detail about diagnosis and management of germ cell tumors.	436, 439, 450 (373, 376, 387)	291, 381	Feb 13
2. Describe the complications of ovarian tumors. How would you diagnose and manage a case of twisted ovarian cyst?	445 (382)	298	-
3. What are the causes of chronic pelvic pain? Describe the clinical features and diagnosis of pelvic endometriosis.	465, 413 (457, 468)	306, 557	-
SHORT NOTES			
1. Differential diagnosis cystic tumors of ovary.	437 (374)	291	-
2. Germ cell tumors of ovary.	439 (376)	381	-
3. Dermoid cyst of ovary (4).	439 (376)	293	Aug 13
4. Dermoid cyst (3).	439 (376)	293	Feb 15
5. Meigs' syndrome.	439 (376)	296, 652	-
6. Solid teratoma of ovary.	440 (377)	383	-
7. Dysgerminoma (6).	441 (378)	381	-
8. Dysgerminoma of ovary (5).	441 (378)	381	Feb 14
9. Granulosa cell tumor (3).	442 (379)	384	Feb 12
10. Complications of ovarian tumors.	445 (382)	298	-

11.	Twisted ovarian cyst (2).	445 (382)	298	-
12.	Galactorrhea.	456 (478)	576	-
13.	Spasmodic dysmenorrhea.	471 (294)	178	-
14.	Congestive dysmenorrhea.	471 (294)	181	-
15.	Dysmenorrhea (2).	471 (294)	178	-
16.	Premenstrual syndrome.	473 (296)	182	-

SHORT ANSWERS

1.	Pseudomyxoma peritonei—causes and prevention.	437 (375)	300	-
2.	Granulosa cell tumor.	442 (379)	384	Aug 15
3.	List the hormone-producing ovarian tumors.	442 (379)	384	-
4.	Complications of ovarian cyst.	445 (382)	299	-
5.	Carcinoembryonic antigen (CEA).	450 (387)	521	-
6.	Ovarian remnant syndrome.	452 (388)	559	-
7.	Gynecological causes for low backache.	468 (-)	561	-
8.	Classification of congestive dysmenorrhea. Mention two causes.	471 (294)	181	-
9.	Spasmodic dysmenorrhea.	471 (294)	178	-
10.	Premenstrual syndrome.	473 (296)	182	Aug 12
11.	Colpotomy.	- (-)	176	Feb 13

Chapters 37 to 40

37. Vulvar and Vaginal Cancer
38. Cervical Intraepithelial Neoplasia, Carcinoma Cervix
39. Cancers of Endometrium, Uterus and Fallopian tube
40. Ovarian Cancer

ESSAYS

	SHW	DUTTA	Recent Years
1. a. What are the causes of postmenopausal bleeding? b. What are the risk factors for development of carcinoma cervix? c. Discuss histological types, symptoms, signs, staging and diagnosis of carcinoma cervix. d. Brief on management of carcinoma (CA) cervix stage I.	76, 485, 495 (71, 399, 407)	559, 322, 340	Feb 14
2. What is CIN*? Discuss in detail the grades, diagnosis and treatment of CIN.	486 (400)	320	Feb 12
3. Discuss the pathology, clinical features and management of endometrial carcinoma (2).	507 (416)	354	–
4. What are the predisposing factors, diagnosis, staging and management of endometrial carcinoma?	507 (416)	354	Aug 11
5. Describe the clinical features, diagnosis and treatment of choriocarcinoma.	513 (258)	362, 383	–
6. Discuss FIGO† staging and management of ovarian carcinoma.	526 (427)	373	Aug 14

*CIN, cervical intraepithelial neoplasia; †FIGO, Federation of Gynecology and Obstetrics.

7.	Describe the staging of malignant ovarian tumors. Discuss its clinical features and management (3)?	526 (427)	373	-

SHORT NOTES

1.	Cervical intraepithelial neoplasia.	486 (400)	320	Aug 12, Feb 13
2.	Classification of CIN and its management (2).	486 (400)	320	-
3.	Carcinoma in situ.	486 (400)	320	-
4.	Screening of carcinoma cervix (4).	488 (402)	324	Aug 11
5.	Early detection of carcinoma cervix.	488 (402)	324	-
6.	Indications of conization of cervix.	489 (-)	326	Aug 13
7.	Laser in gynecology.	491, 173 (327, 394)	123	-
8.	Large loop excision of transformation zone (LLETZ).	493 (406)	328	Feb 14
9.	Symptoms and signs of carcinoma cervix.	497 (409)	344	-
10.	Stages of carcinoma cervix (2).	501 (412)	342	-
11.	Management of cancer cervix.	501 (413)	346	Feb 15
12.	Fractional curettage (4).	510 (419)	357	-
13.	Staging and treatment of choriocarcinoma.	516 (260)	364	Aug 14
14.	Tumor markers (2).	523 (424)	521, 377	-
15.	Arrhenoblastoma.	524 (425)	386	-

SHORT ANSWERS

1.	Indications of per rectal (PR) examination in gynecology.	86 (82)	107	-
2.	Clinical features of carcinoma cervix.	497 (409)	344	-
3.	Predisposing factors for endometrial carcinoma.	507 (416)	354	Aug 12
4.	Fractional curettage.	510 (419)	357	-
5.	Mode of death in carcinoma cervix.	- (-)	346	-

Chapters 41 to 45

	SHW	DUTTA	Recent Years
SHORT NOTES			
1. Chemoradiation.	532 (434)	523, 510	Feb 12
SHORT ANSWERS			
1. Danazol.	551 (313)	530, 311	Feb 13
2. Ovarian hyperstimulation syndrome.	552 (315)	529	-
3. Bromocriptine.	559 (320)	471	Feb 12
4. Cabergoline.	559 (320)	471	Feb 15

BIBLIOGRAPHY

1. Padubidri VG, Daftary SN. Howkins & Bourne Shaw's Textbook of Gynaecology, 16th edition. New Delhi: Reed Elsevier India Private Limited; 2015.
2. Hiralal Konar. DC Dutta's Textbook of Gynaecology, 6th edition. New Delhi: Jaypee Brothers Medical Publishers (P) Ltd; 2013.
3. Hiralal Konar. DC Dutta's Textbook of Obstetrics, 8th edition. New Delhi: Jaypee Brothers Medical Publishers (P) Ltd; 2015.

Section 6

PEDIATRICS

Pediatrics

INSTRUCTIONS TO READERS

- Chapterwise based on OP Ghai's ESSENTIAL PAEDIATRICS, 8th edition (Code: GHAI) with page numbers of answers
- The year in which questions have recently appeared (last nine question papers from Aug 2011 to Aug 2015) have been mentioned under the recent year's heading
- The number of times a question has been repeated between 1990 and 2015, is mentioned within brackets along with the respective questions

Chapters 1 to 7

1. Introduction to Pediatrics
2. Normal Growth and its Disorders
3. Development
4. Adolescent Health and Development
5. Fluid and Electrolyte Disturbances
6. Nutrition
7. Micronutrients in Health and Disease

ESSAYS

	GHAI	Recent Years
1. Enumerate the factors affecting the growth and development in the postnatal period. Discuss the growth and development of a 1-year-old child.	7, 42, 9, 45	–
2. Describe the growth and development of a child up to 2 years of age.	10, 45	–
3. Describe the growth chart. Discuss the uses of growth chart in pediatric clinic and causes of growth failure.	13	–
4. Define dwarfism. Differential diagnosis for dwarfism in a 12-year-old female child.	35	–

5.	Define failure to thrive in children. List the investigations for a 6-month-old baby with failure to thrive. Indicate how to treat a 9-month-old baby with failure to thrive due to faulty feeding technique.	38	–
6.	Classify malnutrition. Describe the clinical features, management and follow-up of malnutrition.	95, 98, 100	Feb 13
7.	How will you identify and evaluate a child with severe acute malnutrition? How will you manage? Discuss the complications and prevention.	97	Aug 15
8.	Describe clinical features of protein-energy malnutrition (PEM). Outline the investigations to be done and its management and complications (2).	99	–
9.	Classify PEM. Outline the clinical features, investigations and management of a 4-year-old child weighing 7 kg with marasmus.	95, 99, 100	–
10.	Enumerate the clinical features of kwashiorkor. Outline the management of a 1-year-old child with severe malnutrition.	99, 101	–
11.	Describe the clinical features, diagnosis and management of nutritional rickets.	113	–

SHORT NOTES

1.	What are the factors that influence growth and development?	7, 42	–
2.	Hormonal influence on growth.	7	–
3.	Radiological assessment of age.	11	–
4.	Temporary dentition.	11	–
5.	Mid-arm circumference.	12, 97	–
6.	Growth charts (2).	13	Feb 13
7.	Road to health charts.	13	–
8.	Short stature.	35	–
9.	Differential diagnosis for short stature.	35	–
10.	Proportionate short stature.	35	Aug 12
11.	Importance of milestone in pediatric practice.	45	–

12.	Milestones of development.	45	–
13.	Developmental screening scales.	55	Feb 14
14.	Adverse effects of television (TV) viewing in children.	57	–
15.	Behavioral disorders in children.	57	Aug 15
16.	Pica in children.	58	–
17.	Breath-holding spell (5).	58	Aug 13
18.	Temper tantrums (2).	58	–
19.	Learning disability.	60	–
20.	Autistic disorder.	61	–
21.	Five stages of sexual maturity rating in girls.	64	–
22.	Psychological problems of adolescent.	65	–
23.	Adolescent vaccines.	69	–
24.	Hypokalemia in children and its management.	76	–
25.	Hypocalcemia—clinical features and management in neonates and children.	80, 180	Aug 15
26.	Acidosis.	85	–
27.	Weaning (4).	91	–
28.	Age-independent anthropometric measurements.	97	Aug 14
29.	Severe acute malnutrition (SAM).	97	–
30.	Marasmus (3).	99	–
31.	Differences between kwashiorkor and marasmus (2).	99	–
32.	ICDS* program (2).	109	Feb 13
33.	Vitamin A deficiency.	111	Feb 13
34.	Signs, symptoms and management of vitamin A deficiency in children.	111	–
35.	Treatment schedule of xerophthalmia.	111	–
36.	Vitamin A prophylaxis (2).	111	–
37.	Xerosis.	111	–
38.	Clinical features of nutritional rickets.	113	–
39.	Nutritional rickets (2).	113	Aug 12
40.	X-ray findings of active rickets.	113	–
41.	Vitamin D-resistant rickets.	114	Aug 14

*ICDS, integrated child development services.

42.	Non-nutritional rickets.	115	–
43.	Zinc deficiency in children.	121	–
44.	Clinical features of zinc deficiency.	121	–
45.	Grading of marasmus.	–	–
46.	Dental caries.	–	–

SHORT ANSWERS

1.	Name the ossification centers present in full term newborn babies.	11	–
2.	Bone age.	11	Aug 12
3.	Bangle test.	97	Aug 13
4.	Differences between breath-holding spell and cyanotic spell.	58, 421	–
5.	Attention deficit hyperactivity disorder (ADHD).	59	Feb 14
6.	Adolescent problems.	65	Feb 12
7.	Vaccines in adolescent period.	69	Aug 12
8.	What are the two key signs of dehydration?	73	–
9.	Electrocardiogram (ECG) changes in hypokalemia.	77	–
10.	Diagnosis and treatment of hyperkalemia.	78	Aug 12
11.	Management of hyperkalemia.	78	Aug 14
12.	Role of dietary fibers in nutrition.	88	Aug 15
13.	Diet chart for 1-year-old child.	89	Aug 12
14.	Four essential features of kwashiorkor.	99	–
15.	ICDS.	109	Aug 14
16.	Vitamin A.	111	–
17.	Vitamin A prophylaxis (3).	111	–
18.	Vitamin A deficiency in children.	111	Feb 12
19.	Treatment of nutritional rickets.	113	–
20.	Management of nutritional rickets.	113	Feb 15
21.	Vitamin K in newborn.	117	–
22.	Role of zinc in children.	121	Aug 15
23.	Clinical features of zinc deficiency.	121	–
24.	Amylase-rich food.	–	–
25.	Features of nutritional recovery syndrome.	–	–

Chapters 8

8. Newborn Infants

ESSAYS

	GHAI	Recent Years
1. Define preterm. Enumerate the causes of preterm. What are the principles in the management of preterm baby?	155	–
2. Define and mention the causes of prematurity. Write about the hazards of premature baby. Mention the care given to a preterm baby of weight 1.6 kg.	155	–
3. Write an essay on etiology, complications and management of preterm baby.	155	–
4. Define normal term baby, preterm baby, low-birth-weight (LBW) baby, intrauterine growth restriction (IUGR) baby. Describe in detail the care of preterm baby in hospital and at home.	155	Feb 12
5. Define prematurity. Discuss the complications of prematurity. How will you manage hyaline membrane disease?	155, 156, 169	Aug 14
6. What are the causes of sepsis in newborn period? Discuss the management and prevention of sepsis in newborn.	163	–
7. Enumerate the causes of respiratory distress in newborn in the first 24 hours of life. Discuss the diagnosis, management and complications of meconium aspiration syndrome (MAS).	169, 170	Aug 12
8. Describe the etiology, pathophysiology and management of MAS.	170	–
9. Clinical features, investigations and management of day 1 jaundice in newborn.	172	–

10.	Define jaundice. What are the common causes of neonatal jaundice? How do you investigate and treat a neonate of 20 days with conjugate hyperbilirubinemia?	172	–
11.	What are the causes of jaundice in the newborn period? How do you investigate and manage a case of Rh incompatibility?	172	–

SHORT NOTES

1.	Exclusive breastfeeding.	134	–
2.	Moro reflex.	142	–
3.	Non-shivering thermogenesis.	143	–
4.	Hypothermia of newborn.	145	–
5.	Kangaroo mother care.	148	–
6.	Importance of breastfeeding.	150	–
7.	Advantages of breastfeeding (2).	150	Aug 13
8.	Causes of lactation failure.	152	–
9.	Reflexes associated with breastfeeding (2).	152	Feb 13
10.	Colostrum.	153	–
11.	Steps for successful breastfeeding.	154	–
12.	Etiology of neonatal sepsis.	163	–
13.	Septicemia in newborn.	163	–
14.	Umbilical sepsis.	163	–
15.	Complications of umbilical cord sepsis.	163	–
16.	Birth asphyxia.	166	–
17.	Hypoxic ischemic encephalopathy.	166	–
18.	Respiratory distress syndrome (RDS) in newborn.	169	Aug 13
19.	MAS.	170	Feb 13
20.	Define apnea in newborn—its causes and management.	171	Aug 15
21.	First day jaundice in the newborn.	172	–
22.	Neonatal jaundice.	172	–
23.	Management of hyperbilirubinemia in newborn.	173	–
24.	Phototherapy.	175	–
25.	Phototherapy in newborn.	175	Feb 15

26. Congenital diaphragmatic hernia.	178	–
27. Infant of diabetic mother (2).	181	Aug 14
28. Therapeutic hypothermia.	–	Aug 14
29. Kernicterus.	–	–
30. Hemorrhagic disease of newborn (2).	–	Aug 12
31. Antenatal diagnosis.	–	–

SHORT ANSWERS

1. APGAR* score.	126	Feb 12
2. Contraindication to bag-mask ventilation.	129	–
3. Reasons for poor chest raise during bag-mask ventilation.	130	–
4. Danger signs in young infant.	134	–
5. Umbilical cord care.	134	–
6. Erythema toxicum.	135	–
7. Four common skin problems in pediatrics.	135	–
8. Four minor physiological problems in neonate.	135	–
9. Large for gestational age (LGA).	137	–
10. Caput succedaneum (2).	141	–
11. Cephalhematoma.	141	Aug 12
12. Hypothermia in newborn—prevention.	145	Feb 12
13. Kangaroo mother care (2).	148	–
14. Four factors that can lessen breast milk production.	152	–
15. Indirect markers of neonatal sepsis.	163	–
16. Sepsis screening in newborn.	163	Aug 14
17. Causes of respiratory distress in newborn.	169	–
18. Differences between physiological and pathological jaundice in newborn.	172	–
19. Physiological jaundice in newborn.	172	Feb 12
20. Principles of phototherapy (2).	175	Aug 12
21. Hypoglycemia.	179	–
22. Medical fetal therapy for lung maturity.	–	Aug 15
23. Baby-friendly hospital initiative (BFHI) (2).	–	Feb 12

* APGAR, 'activity, pulse, grimace, appearance, respiration'.

Chapters 9 to 11

9. Immunization and Immunodeficiency
10. Infections and Infestations
11. Diseases of Gastrointestinal System and Liver

ESSAYS

	GHAI	Recent Years
1. List common causes of pyrexia of unknown origin in children. Briefly indicate investigations for a child with prolonged fever for more than 2 weeks. Discuss the specific treatment for 6-year-old child with falciparum malaria.	211, 263	–
2. Mention the common exanthematous fevers that come across in pediatric age group. Discuss clinical features, diagnosis, management and prevention of measles.	212, 213	–
3. Describe the clinical features, complications, prevention and management of tetanus.	247	–
4. How does primary tuberculosis differ from adult tuberculosis?	251	–
5. Discuss the etiology, pathogenesis, clinical features, complications and management of primary complex in children.	251	–
6. What is primary complex? Discuss natural course of primary complex and its manifestations. How will you investigate and manage a child with primary complex (2)?	251	Aug 13
7. Describe the clinical features, investigations and treatment of a child suffering from cerebral malaria.	262	–
8. Discuss the clinical features, diagnosis and management of acute diarrhea in a child of 2 years.	291	–

9.	What is diarrhea? Discuss the etiopathogenesis, complications, investigations and management of acute watery diarrhea with severe dehydration.	291	–
10.	A 2-year-old female child weighing 8.2 kg brought to the health center with the complaints of vomiting and diarrhea. How will you approach the child? Write the management in detail.	292	–
11.	Define fulminant hepatic failure. Describe its clinical presentation, complications and management.	–	Feb 14

SHORT NOTES

1.	Herd immunity.	189	–
2.	Live attenuated vaccines.	189	Aug 12
3.	Live vaccines.	189	Aug 14
4.	Oral polio vaccine (2).	192	–
5.	Measles vaccination (2).	195	–
6.	Hepatitis B vaccination.	196	–
7.	MMR* vaccine (3).	196	–
8.	Varicella vaccine.	197	–
9.	Typhoid vaccine.	197	Feb 13
10.	Pneumococcal vaccine.	199	–
11.	Human papillomavirus (HPV) vaccine.	200	Feb 14
12.	Adverse events following immunization.	204	–
13.	Universal Immunization Program.	205	–
14.	Cold chain.	205	–
15.	Immunization schedule.	206	–
16.	National Immunization Schedule.	206	–
17.	Exanthematous fever.	212	Feb 13
18.	Complications of measles (5).	213	Feb 13
19.	Difference between measles and German measles.	213	–
20.	Eradication of poliomyelitis.	219	–

*MMR, 'measles, mumps, and rubella.'

21.	Hepatitis B infection.	221	Feb 13
22.	Dengue shock syndrome.	227	Feb 12
23.	Acquired immune deficiency syndrome (AIDS) in pediatrics.	229	–
24.	Pediatric HIV* infection (2).	229	Aug 13
25.	Pediatric AIDS.	229	–
26.	Investigation of HIV in a child of 90 days.	234	–
27.	Prevention of mother-to-child transmission in HIV.	235	Aug 14
28.	Prevention of pediatric AIDS.	235	–
29.	Immunization of infant born to HIV-positive mother.	237	–
30.	Emerging viruses.	239	Aug 14
31.	Differences between diphtheria and follicular tonsillitis.	241	–
32.	Whooping cough.	242	–
33.	Diagnosis and management of enteric fever.	243	Aug 15
34.	Neonatal tetanus.	247	–
35.	Primary complex.	251	–
36.	Fate of primary complex.	251	–
37.	A 1-year-old baby with positive Mantoux.	254	–
38.	Mantoux test (2).	254	–
39.	Tuberculin skin test.	254	–
40.	Cerebral malaria.	262	–
41.	Blackwater fever.	–	–
42.	Toxicity of antimalarial drugs.	264	–
43.	National Malaria Eradication Program.	265	–
44.	Common helminthic infections of childhood.	273	–
45.	Ascariasis (2).	274	–
46.	Gastroesophageal reflux.	280	Aug 12
47.	Management of constipation in children.	283	Aug 14
48.	Gastrointestinal causes of abdominal pain in children.	286	Feb 13
49.	Acute diarrheal disease in 1-year-old child.	291	–
50.	Oral rehydration therapy (3).	294	–

*HIV, human immunodeficiency virus.

51.	Oral rehydration solution (ORS) in acute gastroenteritis (AGE).	294	Feb 12
52.	Chronic diarrhea evaluation and management.	299	Aug 15
53.	Causes of splenomegaly.	310	Feb 14
54.	Causes of acute liver cell failure in children.	313	–
55.	Extrahepatic portal hypertension.	319	Feb 14
56.	Wilson's disease.	320	–
57.	Umbilical hernia.	–	–
58.	Newer vaccines (4).	–	Feb 12
59.	WHO* grading of DHF†.	–	–
60.	Reverse cold chain.	–	Feb 14

SHORT ANSWERS

1.	Indications for intravenous immunoglobulin (Ig) in children.	188	–
2.	Uses of intravenous Ig in pediatrics.	188	Aug 14
3.	Acellular pertussis vaccine.	194	Feb 14
4.	Hepatitis B vaccine schedule.	196	Feb 12
5.	Hepatitis B vaccine.	196	Aug 13
6.	Varicella vaccine.	197	Feb 15
7.	HPV vaccine.	200	–
8.	Antirabies vaccine.	202	Aug 15
9.	Write four common causes of fever with rash.	212	–
10.	Complications of measles.	213	Aug 13
11.	Viral markers for hepatitis B.	221	Feb 15
12.	Prevention of mother-to-child transmission of HIV in HbsAg-positive mothers.	222	Aug 15
13.	Investigations in dengue fever.	226	Feb 12
14.	Name antiretroviral therapy drugs used in HIV-positive pregnant women.	235	–
15.	Prevention of HIV transmission in pediatrics.	235	Feb 12
16.	Write four complications of diphtheria.	242	–
17.	Treatment of pertussis.	243	–

* WHO, World Health Organization; †DHF, dengue hemorrhagic fever.

18.	Diagnosis of leptospirosis.	246	–
19.	Components of primary complex.	251	–
20.	Interferon gamma release assay.	253	Aug 12
21.	Quantitative buffy coat.	262	Feb 13
22.	Falciparum malaria complications.	266	Feb 12
23.	Congenital rubella syndrome.	272	Feb 14
24.	Use of ivermectin.	275	–
25.	Gastroesophageal (GE) reflux in children.	280	Feb 14
26.	Management of acute diarrhea.	291	Aug 12
27.	Oral rehydration therapy corner.	294	–
28.	ORS.	294	Aug 13
29.	Hypo-osmolar ORS.	294	Feb 15
30.	Explain four common causes of persistent diarrhea.	297	–
31.	Chronic causes of diarrhea in children.	300	Feb 12
32.	Clinical features of chronic liver disease.	316	Aug 12
33.	Etiology of cirrhosis.	316	–
34.	Treatment of Wilson's disease.	321	Feb 14
35.	Four newer vaccines.	–	–
36.	Reverse cold chain.	–	Feb 12
37.	Newer antimalarial drugs.	–	Feb 12
38.	Shake test.	–	–

Chapters 12 to 15

12. Hematological Disorders
13. Otolaryngology
14. Disorders of Respiratory System
15. Disorders of Cardiovascular System

ESSAYS

		GHAI	Recent Years
1.	What are the stages of red blood corpuscles? What are the clinical features, laboratory investigations and management of nutritional anemia in a child (iron deficiency).	330, 334	–
2.	Discuss the causes and clinical features of anemia of infancy. Briefly discuss the management of thalassemia major.	331, 342	–
3.	What are the common causes of acute bronchiolitis? How do you investigate and manage a child of 9 months with severe distress?	381	–
4.	Discuss the common causes, clinical features, management and prevention of acute respiratory infection in children.	–	
5.	Describe etiology, pathophysiology, clinical features and management of congestive cardiac failure in children (2).	396	–
6.	Classify congenital heart diseases. Discuss the hemodynamic assessment of severity, its course and complications of ventricular septal defect.	400, 414	–
7.	Describe the etiopathogenesis, clinical features, investigations, treatment and prevention of rheumatic fever (2).	434	Feb 13
8.	Define acute rheumatic fever. Mention etiopathogenesis, clinical features and management of rheumatic carditis.	434	–

9.	How would you treat a case of acute rheumatic fever with carditis? Discuss the prognosis of such a case.	437	–
10.	Discuss the etiology, pathogenesis, clinical features, investigations and management of acute rheumatic fever in children. Mention complications and the prevention of acute rheumatic fever.	437	Feb 15
11.	Discuss etiopathogenesis and clinical manifestations of rheumatic mitral stenosis.	440	–

SHORT NOTES

1.	Peripheral smear study in diagnosis of hematological disorders.	332	Feb 12
2.	Difference between iron deficiency anemia and hemolytic anemia.	334,337	–
3.	Peripheral smear in thalassemia.	341	–
4.	Thalassemia major.	341	–
5.	Management of thalassemia.	342	Feb 14
6.	Sickle cell crisis.	344	Aug 12
7.	Acute idiopathic thrombocytopenia purpura (ITP).	351	–
8.	ITP (2).	351	Aug 13
9.	Complications of otitis media.	361	–
10.	Differential diagnosis for child with epistaxis.	373	–
11.	Pneumonia.	377	–
12.	Staphylococcal pneumonia.	378	Aug 12
13.	Atypical pneumonia in children.	379	–
14.	Acute respiratory tract infection (ARI) control program (2).	380	Feb 12
15.	Acute bronchiolitis.	381	–
16.	Management of status asthmaticus.	390	–
17.	Status asthmaticus.	390	–
18.	Components of Kartagener's syndrome.	392	–
19.	Signs, symptoms and management of idiopathic RDS in a newborn.	393	–

20.	Prevention and management of RDS in newborn.	393	Feb 15
21.	Differential diagnosis of a 1-year-old child with acute respiratory distress and management.	393	Feb 12
22.	Management of congestive cardiac failure.	396	–
23.	Management of cardiac failure.	396	Aug 12
24.	Fallot's tetralogy (3).	420	–
25.	Anoxic spells.	421	–
26.	Cyanotic spells (6).	421	–
27.	Management of cyanotic spell.	421	Feb 15
28.	Eisenmenger's syndrome.	428	–
29.	Acute rheumatic carditis.	434	–
30.	Acute rheumatic fever.	434	–
31.	Rheumatic fever (2).	434	–
32.	Rheumatic fever prophylaxis.	438	–
33.	Treatment of infective endocarditis.	445	Feb 12
34.	Infective endocarditis prophylaxis.	446	–
35.	Differential diagnosis of cervical lymphadenitis.	–	–
36.	Jugular venous pulse.	–	–

SHORT ANSWERS

1.	Physiological anemia of infancy.	331	Aug 12
2.	Peripheral smear in iron deficiency anemia (2).	334	Aug 13
3.	Diagnosis of iron deficiency anemia.	334	Feb 13
4.	Microcytic hypochromic anemia.	334	Aug 14
5.	Peripheral blood picture in thalassemia major.	341	–
6.	Diagnosis of thalassemia.	341	Feb 15
7.	Vascular causes for bleeding.	351	–
8.	Oral candidiasis.	366	Aug 12
9.	Treatment of streptococcal pharyngitis.	367	–
10.	Common causes of wheezing in children.	372	Feb 13
11.	Exercise-induced asthma.	383	Feb 13
12.	Stepwise management of bronchial asthma.	384	–
13.	Leukotriene modifiers.	385	Aug 14

14.	Management of acute severe asthma.	390	Aug 13
15.	Clinical features of empyema thoracis.	395	Feb 13
16.	Types of ventricular septal defect (VSD).	414	–
17.	Common causes of childhood hypertension.	451	Aug 12
18.	Innocent systolic murmurs.	–	Aug 13

Chapters 16 to 19

16. Disorders of Kidney and Urinary Tract
17. Endocrine and Metabolic Disorders
18. Central Nervous System
19. Neuromuscular Disorders

ESSAYS

		GHAI	Recent Years
1.	Mention differential diagnosis in a 4 years child with gross hematuria. Define and classify acute glomerulonephritis. Write clinical features and management of acute poststreptococcal glomerulonephritis.	471, 474	–
2.	Describe the etiology, clinical manifestations and management of acute glomerulonephritis in children.	474	–
3.	A 4-year-old child has been brought to the hospital with swollen face and limbs. Enumerate the causes. What investigations are to be done? Discuss the management of nephrotic syndrome.	477	–
4.	Define nephrotic syndrome. Describe the etiology, clinical features, laboratory investigations and management of minimal change nephrotic syndrome (2).	477	–
5.	Describe the etiology, pathology, clinical features, diagnosis, complications, investigations and management of childhood nephrotic syndrome (4).	477	Aug 14
6.	What are the causes of proportionate dwarfism? Describe the features of endemic goiter and also investigations and treatments for the same.	35, 512, 519	–
7.	Define seizure? What are the common causes of neonatal seizures? How will you investigate and treat a neonate of 10 days old with seizures?	552	–

8.	Describe the etiology, investigations and management of newborn presenting with seizures.	553	–
9.	What are the common causes of convulsion in a 1-year-old febrile infant? Outline the management.	556	–
10.	Discuss the differential diagnosis for a child of 1 year age brought with history of fever, unconsciousness, convulsions to the hospital. How will you proceed with the management of ill child?	556	Feb 12
11.	A 9-month-old infant comes to the hospital with fever and altered sensorium. List out the causes. How will you investigate the case? Discuss the management of acute bacterial meningitis.	563	–
12.	Describe the clinical features, diagnosis, management and complications of acute bacterial meningitis in children.	563	Feb 14
13.	Describe the etiopathogenesis, clinical features, complications and management of bacterial meningitis.	563	Aug 12
14.	Discuss the etiopathogenesis, clinical features, diagnosis and management of tuberculous (TB) meningitis in children (2).	566	–
15.	What are the etiology, clinical features, diagnostic techniques, complications and management of acute meningitis in infants?	563	–
16.	Describe briefly CSF* circulation. Discuss the etiology, clinical features and management of hydrocephalus in a newborn baby (2).	574	–
17.	Discuss the differential diagnosis of an infant with a large head. Outline signs and symptoms of hydrocephalus in infancy and children.	40, 574	Aug 13
18.	Define cerebral palsy. Discuss the etiopathogenesis, types, management and differential diagnosis of cerebral palsy.	581	–

*CSF, cerebrospinal fluid.

19. Discuss the etiology, clinical features and differential diagnosis of the common causes of acute flaccid paralysis in children. Outline the management of conditions.	592	-
20. A 8-month-old infant is brought with history of weakness of right lower limb with fever of 5 days. Discuss the diagnosis, complications and management.	592	-
21. Discuss the clinical manifestations, diagnosis and management of acute leukemias of childhood.	599	-

SHORT NOTES

1. Urine examination.	468	-
2. Urine examination in nephritis and nephrotic syndrome.	474, 477	-
3. Poststreptococcal glomerulonephritis.	474	Feb 14
4. Complications and management of acute glomerulonephritis.	474	Feb 15
5. Minimal change nephrotic syndrome.	477	-
6. Nephrotic syndrome (4).	477	-
7. Renal biopsy in nephrotic syndrome, and indications and contraindications of the same.	478	Feb 12
8. Management of acute renal failure.	487	Aug 13
9. Causes and management of enuresis in children.	504	-
10. Nocturnal enuresis.	504	Aug 14
11. Posterior urethral valves.	506	-
12. Congenital hypothyroidism (2).	516	Aug 13
13. Cretin (4).	519	-
14. Cushing's syndrome.	523	-
15. Childhood obesity.	528	Aug 12
16. Causes of convulsions in newborn period (2).	553	Aug 13
17. Status epilepticus (2).	553	-
18. Phenobarbitone in pediatric practice.	554	-
19. Febrile seizures (4).	556	Feb 12

20. Management of febrile fits.	556	–
21. Difference between febrile convulsion and convulsion due to meningitis.	556	–
22. Infantile spasms.	559	–
23. Management of pyogenic meningitis in a 1-year-old infant.	563	–
24. Pyogenic meningitis.	563	–
25. CSF findings in TB meningitis (2).	567	–
26. Diagnosis of TB meningitis (2).	567	Aug 13
27. Reye's syndrome (2).	569	–
28. Hydrocephalus.	574	Feb 14
29. Pseudotumor cerebri (2).	575	Aug 12
30. Common metabolic neuropathies.	590	–
31. Acute flaccid paralysis surveillance.	219, 592	–
32. Alpha-fetoprotein (AFP).	592	–
33. Duchenne muscular dystrophy (2).	595	Feb 14

SHORT ANSWERS

1. DMSA* scan.	470	Feb 14
2. Important causes of hematuria.	471	–
3. Write four clinical features of acute glomerulonephritis.	474	–
4. Definition of nephrotic syndrome.	477	–
5. Complications of nephrotic syndrome.	480	Feb 14
6. Steroid toxicity.	481	–
7. Diagnosis of UTI.	484	Feb 13
8. Vesicoureteral reflux.	485	Aug 14
9. Write four clinical features of hypothyroidism.	516	–
10. Neonatal screening for hypothyroidism.	517	–
11. Cryptorchidism.	540	Aug 12
12. Signs and symptoms of diabetic ketoacidosis.	547	Feb 13
13. Neuroimaging.	551	Aug 14
14. Management of status epilepticus.	553	Feb 14
15. Common organisms causing meningitis.	563	–

*DMSA, dimercaptosuccinic acid.

16.	Stages of TB meningitis.	566	Feb 13
17.	CSF findings in TB meningitis.	567	Feb 14
18.	Causes of acquired hydrocephalus.	574	-
19.	Pseudotumor cerebri causes.	575	-
20.	Early indicators of cerebral palsy.	582	Aug 12
21.	Causes of preventable mental retardation (2).	585	-

Chapters 20 to 31

20. Childhood Malignancies
21. Rheumatological Disorders
22. Genetic Disorders
23. Inborn Errors of Metabolism
24. Eye Disorders
25. Skin Disorders
26. Poisoning, Injuries and Accidents
27. Pediatric Critical Care
28. Common Medical Procedures
29. Rational Drug Therapy
30. Integrated Management of Neonatal and Childhood Illness
31. Rights of Children

ESSAYS

		GHAI	Recent Years
1.	Discuss the clinical manifestations, diagnosis and management of acute leukemia of childhood.	599	–

SHORT NOTES

		GHAI	Recent Years
1.	Acute lymphatic leukemia (2).	599	Aug 13
2.	Diagnosis of acute leukemia.	601	Feb 12
3.	Down syndrome (4).	637	–
4.	Genetics of Down syndrome.	638	Feb 14
5.	Antenatal diagnosis of Down syndrome.	638	Feb 15
6.	Neonatal screening.	645	Aug 14
7.	Genetic counseling (2).	646	–
8.	Scabies in children (3).	694	–
9.	Treatment of salicylate intoxication.	701	–
10.	Steps in treatment in organophosphorus (OPC) poisoning.	701	–
11.	Kerosene poisoning (3).	702	–
12.	Scorpion sting.	703	–
13.	Snake envenomation.	703	–
14.	Platelet transfusion.	724	–

15. Indications for bone marrow examination in children.	736	–
16. Cephalosporins.	741	–
17. Give five basic rights of child.	768	–
18. Reproductive and child health (RCH) program (4).	–	–
19. Baby-friendly hospital initiative (2).	–	–
20. Birth injuries.	–	–
21. Infant mortality rate (2).	–	–

SHORT ANSWERS

1. Classification of acute lymphoblastic leukemia (ALL).	600	Feb 13
2. Chemotherapy in ALL.	603	Aug 12
3. Juvenile rheumatoid arthritis.	625	–
4. Ultrasonography (USG) findings of Down syndrome antenatally.	639	–
5. X-linked inheritance.	641	Aug 14
6. Galactosemia.	655	Aug 13
7. Digoxin toxicity.	701	Aug 13
8. Management of snake bite.	703	Feb 12
9. Features of viper envenomation.	703	–
10. Scorpion sting.	703	Feb 12
11. Types of shock (2).	715	Feb 13
12. Importance of bone marrow examination.	736	Feb 14
13. Triple test in newborn screening.	–	–
14. RCH.	–	Aug 13
15. Infant mortality rate.	–	Aug 14

BIBLIOGRAPHY

1. Ghai OP. Essential Pediatrics, 8th edition. New Delhi: CBS Publishers & Distributors; 2013.